PARASITES AND PARASITIC DISEASES

Edited by **Gilberto Bastidas**

Parasites and Parasitic Diseases
http://dx.doi.org/10.5772/intechopen.73726
Edited by Gilberto Bastidas

Contributors

Greanious Alfred Mavondo, Obadiah Moyo, Joy Mavondo, Mary Dlodlo, Wisdom Peresu, Jose Luis Muñoz-Carrillo, Alejandra Moreno-García, Juan Armando Flores-De La Torre, José Jesús Muñoz-Escobedo, Argelia López-Luna, Claudia Maldonado-Tapia, Gaoussou Coulibaly, John Kagira, John Mokua, David Kamau, Naomi Maina, Maina Ngotho, Adele Njuguna, Simon Karanja, Lucy Mutharia, Gilberto Antonio Bastidas Pacheco

Notice

Statements and opinions expressed in the chapters are these of the individual contributors and not necessarily those of the editors or publisher. No responsibility is accepted for the accuracy of information contained in the published chapters. The publisher assumes no responsibility for any damage or injury to persons or property arising out of the use of any materials, instructions, methods or ideas contained in the book.

First published in London, United Kingdom, 2019 by IntechOpen
IntechOpen is the global imprint of INTECHOPEN LIMITED, registered in England and Wales, registration number: 11086078, The Shard, 25th floor, 32 London Bridge Street
London, SE19SG – United Kingdom
Printed in Croatia

British Library Cataloguing-in-Publication Data
A catalogue record for this book is available from the British Library

Additional hard copies can be obtained from orders@intechopen.com

Parasites and Parasitic Diseases, Edited by Gilberto Bastidas
p. cm.
Print ISBN 978-1-83880-127-4
Online ISBN 978-1-83880-128-1

We are IntechOpen,
the world's leading publisher of Open Access books
Built by scientists, for scientists

4,100+
Open access books available

116,000+
International authors and editors

120M+
Downloads

Our authors are among the

151
Countries delivered to

Top 1%
most cited scientists

12.2%
Contributors from top 500 universities

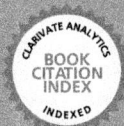

CLARIVATE ANALYTICS
BOOK CITATION INDEX
INDEXED

WEB OF SCIENCE™

Selection of our books indexed in the Book Citation Index
in Web of Science™ Core Collection (BKCI)

Interested in publishing with us?
Contact book.department@intechopen.com

Numbers displayed above are based on latest data collected.
For more information visit www.intechopen.com

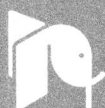

Meet the editor

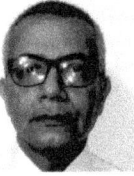

Gilberto Bastidas is a medical surgeon graduate from the University of the Andes, with diplomas in prehospital emergency care, executive management for senior management in health, and health and safety at work. He also has a health management course equivalent to a medium course in public health and an MSc in Education Management and Protozoology. He is a doctor in parasitology. In the research field, Dr. Bastidas is the author of several articles published in national and international journals and has served as arbitrator for scientific articles. He is part of the editorial committee of several national and international journals, a textbook writer, and a lecturer. Nowadays, he is classified as PEII level C in the government program to stimulate the Venezuelan researcher.

Contents

Preface

The main idea of this book is to collect information on parasitology as a biological science. One particular branch of ecology of particular interest in this book is parasitism, which is understood to be the relationship between parasite, host, and environment. These aspects are related to life cycle, clinical manifestations, immune response, evasion and adaptation mechanisms, diagnosis, treatment, and epidemiology.

It is therefore a text that serves as a reference to students and professionals of health sciences in their clinical practice. It centers on animal and human parasitic diseases, to promote and protect health and cure or relieve symptoms when it is not possible to eliminate infections. This small compendium shares data from recent research in the field of parasitic diseases.

It also serves as a stimulus for researchers to encourage them to publish or make their work available to others. In this way, their work is projected in the field of research, and financial and academic support is provided so that they can promote their ideas, projects, or research plans.

Gilberto Bastidas
Department of Public Health and Center for Medical and Biotechnological Research
Faculty of Health Sciences
University of Carabobo, Venezuela

Introductory Chapter: Parasitology and Parasitism Areas of Knowledge That Must Be Constantly Studied

Bastidas Gilberto

Additional information is available at the end of the chapter

http://dx.doi.org/10.5772/intechopen.85181

1. Parasitology and parasitism

Parasitology, an important part of biology, is the science responsible for the study of parasitism, that is, the relationship between parasite, host, and environment, in the understanding that parasite is that living being that is housed and/or fed by another living being during part or all of its life, generally who is staying is of different species, of greater size, and more developed structure than the host; the parasite is understood. The relationship between living beings is complex; therefore, the study of it must be constant and from different approaches, with the purpose of increasing and deepening knowledge about it [1]. So:

> Parasitism is a form of ecological interaction, in which a member, the parasite, benefits from the use of resources gathered by another member, the host. Through its evolutionary history, the species have coexisted with populations of parasites that have regulated, along with other ecological interactions, both their sizes and their population structures and their genetic structure. Parasites have an influence on hosts, similar to that of predators, competitors and other natural enemies. In fact, the influence of a parasite on a host can affect its response to competitors and mutualists, its reaction to the physical conditions of the environment, its state of health, its reproductive capacity, its ability to obtain resources or its conservation. The essence of parasitism rests on the parasite-host interaction [2]. Thus:

> "The essence of parasitism is based on the nature of the parasitic-host relationship, that an ecological definition is the study of the relationships between the organism and its environment. However, ecologically the parasite-host relationship is a 'double-edged sword.' Because the ecology of the host can be considered simultaneously in the life cycle of a parasite, in such a way that the host is the habitat for the parasite. Many of the biotic and abiotic variants influence the ecology of the hosts, also affecting the parasite" [3].

That is why the relationship between living beings is complex; therefore, the study of it must be constant and from different approaches, with the purpose of increasing and deepening knowledge about it. This is particularly relevant for the complex biological cycles that parasites follow in their lives (in search of temperature, humidity, and food conducive to live, reproduce, and perpetuate the species), often marked by different evolutionary forms and reproductive or maturation stage, which also implies the passage through more than one host in many of these species and even with different degrees of specificity, ranging from those restricted to a single host species to those capable of developing into host species very far phylogenetically [4].

The foregoing highlights the universality and complexity of the health problems caused by the different species of parasites that affect communities in all countries of the world and reveals the dedication of a large number of academics dedicated to basic, clinical, and epidemiological research in pursuit of control or eradication of them [4].

Parasitology seeks to unravel, the purpose of this book, the dynamic process that is established between parasite and host, in terms of molecular matrix, parasitic adaptation, modifications induced by the host, pathogenesis, clinical manifestations, diagnosis, and treatment, among other aspects, as well as already within the vast field of ecology, the vital conditions, and the environment of obligatory or facultative parasitism, that is, protozoa, helminths, or arthropods, be monoxenous or heteroxenous parasites, both at the individual and population level [5].

The writing of this document encourages the fact that parasitic diseases are not considered as important public health problems, or as a cause of epidemiological emergencies, and because the poor and poorly served populations are the most affected, also those that do not invest enough in research of new therapeutic and diagnostic tools, because they are considered in many cases not very lucrative. This is despite the fact that parasitism is one of the most widespread lifestyles in nature, it is pointed out that practically any living organism can host some kind of parasite [6].

The sure thing is that parasitism implies some degree of loss of biological efficiency in the host that result in slight to severe damage to its structure, which of course justifies its inclusion among the great aspects or issues to be considered in biology, in the medical, and veterinary research within the framework of the great biodiversity, which are the point of origin of the approach to such fascinating life forms, perhaps one of the most striking in nature, this is particularly interesting due to the fact that parasitic diseases. The intensity, period of appearance, age groups, and even sex affect human and animal differently [7–9].

To this it is added that parasites are not kept confined in the regions where they are generally endemic, since it is known that due to incidental or accidental circumstances, these can be transported to other regions to which they can adapt and produce infections and diseases in the populations of animals and humans living there; therefore, the updating of the epidemiological behavior (always complex and dynamic) by specialists in the field is absolutely necessary and indispensable for effective intervention against its spread, or spread reduces the impact they have on animal and human welfare [10, 11].

Parasitic diseases are currently considered a serious public health problem around the world, of course, with more severe consequences in countries with less economic development and of course in the poor and rural areas of most of the countries that make up the region. In planet Earth, to the point that the incidence and prevalence of parasitic diseases are considered as indicators of the health status of animal and human populations and the conditions in which they live, for example, in Latin America, the prevalence of parasitic diseases is persistently elevated, perhaps due to dynamic processes of repeated reinfections, where infection pressure and host susceptibility come into play [12–15].

In summary, etiological agents, biological cycles, and the processes of invasion, establishment, and propagation should be constantly reviewed, as well as the mechanisms of defense and evasion and of pathogenesis, in order to elucidate or at least try the complex parasite–host relationship, and offer a better understanding of the clinical manifestations that consent to laying the rational basis for the control of parasite. With the inescapable consideration of the epidemiological aspects, that allow to answer the where, when and why of the appearance of parasitic diseases and of the risk factors involved in the genesis of them and contribute with this in the policies and designs of effective interventions to modify the adverse health situation, this because despite the great scientific and technological advances in the field of human and veterinary medicine, the parasite, curable and preventable in its majority continue to be a serious threat to health [16, 17].

2. Globalization in the life of the human being: another reason to investigate parasitology

With the globalization of the life of the human being, its technology, its development, trade, and tourism, there has been an impressive increase in the dissemination of diseases generated by parasites, as they are not restricted by geographical barriers, to which enormously sophisticated and modern systems of air, sea, and land transportation are currently available for the movement of humans, animals, and virtually this represents a fundamental reason for the constant study of the epidemiological behavior of parasites in their daily effort to ensure their survival [11].

There are several parasite species capable of producing epidemics, especially through water and food, among which the protozoa, capable of causing giardiasis, cryptosporidiosis, cyclosporiasis, and toxoplasmosis, are favored by these routes of dissemination. Also the increase of immunocompromised individuals due to diseases such as AIDS and changes or combinations of cultural patterns regarding customs and habits in the human groups derived from displacements, for example, the practice of eating foods that are not cooked or raw, which undoubtedly they favor parasitic infection [10, 11, 18–21].

Another factor to mention in the context of globalization as a cause of dissemination of parasitic diseases is the modification that has been made to the environment and that has caused global warming within the so-called climate change that contributes to the spread of diseases transmitted by arthropods, in function of those parasites with forms or evolutionary stages or their life cycle that have a mandatory passage through the earth to complete their life cycle. However, the interconnection that characterizes humanity requires the constant updating of knowledge about parasitic diseases in order to control them and, if possible, eradicate them [11, 22, 23].

Author details

Bastidas Gilberto

Address all correspondence to: bastidasprotozoo@hotmail.com

Department of Public Health and Center for Medical and Biotechnological Research, Faculty of Health Sciences, University of Carabobo, Carabobo State, Venezuela

References

[1] Piekarski G. Lehrbuch der parásitologie. Alemania: Vorschau; 1954

[2] Rico-Hernández G. Evolución de interacciones parásito-hospedero: Coevolución, selección sexual y otras teorías propuestas. Revista U.D.C.A Actualidad & Divulgación Científica. 2011;**14**(2):119-130

[3] Bautista-Hernández C, Monks S, Pulido-Flores G, Rodríguez-Ibarra A. Revisión bibliográfica de algunos términos ecológicos usados en parasitología, y su aplicación en estudios de caso. Estudios de Biodiversidad. 2015;**2**:1-19. University of Nebraska - Lincoln DigitalCommons@University of Nebraska – Lincoln. Available in: http://digitalcommons.unl.edu/biodiversidad/2

[4] Werner L. Parásitología humana. México: McGraw-Hill Interamericana Editores, S.A.; 2013

[5] Brumpt E. Précis de Parásitologie. Paris: Masson; 1913

[6] Naquira C. Las zoonosis parasitarias: Problema de salud pública en el Perú. Revista Peruana de Medicina Experimental y Salud Pública. 2010;**27**(4):494-497

[7] Neghme A, Silva R. Ecología del parasitismo en el hombre. Boletín de la Oficina Sanitaria Panamericana. 1971. Available in: http://iris.paho.org/xmlui/bitstream/handle/123456789/15245/v70n4p313.pdf?sequence=1

[8] Daszak P, Cunningham A, Hyatt A. Emerging infectious diseases of wildlife-threats to biodiversity and human health. Science. 2000;**287**:443-449

[9] Pérez-Tris J. La parasitología ecológica en la era de la genética molecular. Ecosistemas: Revista Cietifica y Tecnica de Ecologia y Medio Ambiente. 2009;**18**(1):52-59. Available in: http://www.revistaecosistemas.net/articulo.asp?Id=596

[10] Macpherson C. Human behavior and the epidemiology of parasitic zoonoses. International Journal for Parasitology. 2005;**35**:1319-1331

[11] Chacin-Bonilla L. Las enfermedades parasitarias intestinales como un problema de salud global. Investigación Clínica. 2013;**54**(1):1-4

[12] Atías A. Parasitología Médica. Mediterráneo: Santiago; 1999

[13] Devera R, Angulo V, Amaro E, Finali M, Franceshi G, Blanco Y, et al. Parásitos intes-
       tinales en habitantes de una comunidad rural del Estado Bolívar, Venezuela. Revista
       Biomedica. 2006;**17**:259-268

[14] Iannacone J, Benites M, Chirinos L. Prevalencia de infección por parásitos intestinales en
       escolares de primaria de Santiago de Surco, Lima, Perú. Parasitología latinoamericana.
       2006;**61**:54-62

[15] Pezzani B, Minvielle M, Ciarmela M, Apezteguía M, Basualdo J. Participación comu-
       nitaria en el control de las parasitosis intestinales en una localidad rural de Argentina.
       Revista Pan American Journal of Public Health (PAJPH). 2009;**26**(6):471-477

[16] Musto A, Bosisio N, Do Nascimento M, Iserte J, Musto A, Orellana M, et al. Manual de
       Microbiología y parasitología. 2da Edición ed. Argentina: Universidad Nacional Arturo
       Jauretche; 2013

[17] Theobald S, Brandes N, Gyapong M, El-Saharty S, Proctor E, Diaz T, et al. Implementation
       research: New imperatives and opportunities in global health. Lancet. 2018;**392**(10160):2214-
       2228. DOI: 10.1016/S0140-6736(18)32205-0

[18] Karanis P, Kourenti C, Smith H. Waterborne transmission of protozoan parasites: A world-
       wide review of outbreaks and lessons learnt. Journal of Water and Health. 2007;**5**:1-38

[19] Jones J, Dubey J. Waterborne toxoplasmosis—Recent developments. Experimental Para-
       sitology. 2010;**124**:10-25

[20] Chacín-Bonilla L, Sánchez-Chávez Y, Estevéz J, Larreal Y, Molero E. Prevalence of
       human toxoplasmosis in the San Carlos Island, Venezuela. Interciencia. 2003;**28**:457-462

[21] Chacín-Bonilla L. Transmission of *Cyclospora cayetanensis* infection: A review focusing
       on soil-borne cyclosporiasis. Transactions of the Royal Society of Tropical Medicine and
       Hygiene. 2008;**102**:215-216

[22] Weaver HJ, Hawdon JM, Hoberg EP. Soil-transmitted helminthiases: Implications of
       climate change and human behavior. Trends in Parasitology. 2010;**26**:574-581

[23] Chacín-Bonilla L. El problema de las parasitosis intestinales en Venezuela. Investigación
       Clínica. 1990;**31**:1-2

Organ Pathology and Associated IFN-γ and IL-10 Variations in Mice Infected with *Toxoplasma gondii* Isolate from Kenya

John Mokua Mose, David Muchina Kamau,
John Maina Kagira, Naomi Maina, Maina Ngotho,
Lucy Mutharia and Simon Muturi Karanja

Additional information is available at the end of the chapter

http://dx.doi.org/10.5772/intechopen.79700

Abstract

Toxoplasma gondii is an important foodborne opportunistic pathogen that causes a severe disease in immunocompromised patients. The pathology and immune responses associated with the ensuing disease have not been well described in strains from different parts of the world. The aim of the present study is to determine the IFN-γ and IL-10 variations and organ pathology in immunocompetent and immunocompromised mice infected with *T. gondii* isolated from a Kenyan chicken. Two groups of BALB/c mice were infected with *T. gondii* cysts and administered with dexamethasone (DXM) in drinking water. Other two groups: infected untreated and uninfected mice were kept as controls. The mice were euthanized at various time points: blood collected for serum and assayed for IFN-γ and IL-10 variations. After infection, significant ($p<0.05$) elevated levels of IFN-γ and IL-10 were observed. A significant decline in IFN-γ and IL-10 levels ($p<0.05$) was observed after dexamethasone treatment. Histological sections in the liver, heart, and spleen of the mice administered with DXM revealed various degrees of inflammation characterized by infiltration of inflammatory cells. The dexamethasone-treated mice presented with progressively increased ($p<0.001$) inflammatory responses is compared with the infected untreated mice.

Keywords: *Toxoplasma gondii*, dexamethasone, IFN-γ, IL-10, organ pathology

1. Introduction

Toxoplasmasmosis, cause by *Toxoplasma gondii*, is rated the most prevalent parasitic zoonotic disease infecting nearly 2 billion people in the world [1]. The infection may be acquired by oral ingestion of food or water contaminated with oocysts present in the feces of members of the cat family, the definitive hosts for *T. gondii*. Other routes of infections include ingestion of tissue cysts found in undercooked meat and congenitally by transplacental transmission [2].

Cases of toxoplasmosis have been reported in Kenya with the earliest study documented in 1968 [3]. Since then, *T. gondii* has been detected in the general Kenyan population as well as susceptible groups with reduced immunity. A serological survey of 127 children revealed a significant rise of prevalence of the *T. gondii*-specific antibodies from 35% in pre-school to 60% in the early school age group [4]. Screening results for blood donors at Kenyatta National Referral Hospital in Nairobi, Kenya indicated high seroprevalence [5]. Fifty four percent (54%) of HIV positive patients attending Kenyatta National Hospital, Nairobi had *Toxoplasma* specific IgG in contrast to 1% of the HIV negative group [6]. A clinical case report of toxoplasmosis was documented in a patient with HIV infection [7]. About 12.7% of hospitalized HIV positive patients with neurological complications at a private hospital in Nairobi, had *T. gondii* infection [8]. Co-infection of *T. gondii* and other parasites such as *Toxocara canis* has been investigated using samples from Kenyans. *Toxoplasma gondii* was detected in five of seven *T. canis*–positive sera from Maasailand [9]. Chunge and colleagues [10] showed that a moderate number of pregnant women attending a Kenyan referral hospital had *T. gondii* antibodies [10]. Such publications and clinical case reports show that there is widespread distribution toxoplamsois in Kenya.

Natural *T. gondii* infection has been detected in free-living and captive animals [11]. Of these 8 of 8 (100%) captive carnivores, 14 of 19 (74%) captive herbivores, 11 of 14 (79%) free-living carnivores and 97 of 118 (82%) free-living herbivores were found to have *Toxoplasma* antibodies. The detection of *Toxoplasma gondii* in free-range chickens is a good indicator of possible risk to human beings. In a study carried out in Thika region, Kenya, the prevalence of *T. gondii* in the chicken was 79.0% indicating high environmental contamination with *T. gondii* oocysts [12]. In another study carried out by Adele et al. [12] in Thika region, *Toxoplasma gondii* oocysts were detected in 7.8% of the cat samples collected. In the same region of Kenya, up to 39% of the slaughterhouse workers were infected with *T. gondii* as detected using nPCR [13]. Several studies have shown the circulation of various strains of *T. gondii* in Kenya, with the most abundant being type II strain [14, 15].

Infection of immunologically competent persons with *T. gondii* most often results in asymptomatic infection where the parasite forms tissue cysts containing bradyzoites in a variety of organs, particularly the brain, heart, and skeletal muscle. However, in immunosuppressed hosts such as those with AIDS, organ transplantation and radiotherapy, there is a high risk for severe infection [16, 17]. In these individuals, the bradyzoite gets reactivated and gets transformed to tachyzoites which cause severe pathology in the heart, liver and spleen [18]. Cellular immunity plays key role in the host's immune reaction against toxoplasmosis [19]. The macrophages and "natural killer" (NK) cells exert their function via a cytotoxic activity and/or the secretion of cytokines involved in the regulation of immune response [20]. *In vivo* studies have shown that IFN-γ is a major cytokine, which is produced by CD4 and CD8 T cells, which mediates resistance against *T. gondii* infection [21]. Thus, IFN-γ is the main type one cytokine involved in toxoplamosis, although other cytokines such as TNF-α, IL-18, IL-22, and the macrophage migration inhibitory factor (MIF) have also been reported in mediating the observed pathology [22]. As the disease progresses, some studies have reported that IL-10 counters the harmful effect of an exaggerated type-1 inflammatory response [23]. From the foregoing, it is clear that the development of a strong cellular immune response is critical for the control of the *T. gondii* infections in the intermediate hosts.

In a study carried out in Kenya, a neurological murine model of chronic toxoplasmosis in BALB/c was developed in BALB/c mice using *T. gondii* isolated from free range chicken [24]. The brain of toxoplasmosis infected mice showed cellular inflammatory infiltrations, neuronal necrosis, and cuffing. Other studies have showed lymphocytes and plasma cells to be the predominant cells in brains of patients having a coinfection of HIV and toxoplasmosis [25]. The severity of pathology was higher in mice immunosuppressed with dexamethasone compared to the control groups. The findings demonstrated that a dexamethasone-induced reactivation of chronic toxoplasmosis may be useful development of laboratory animal model in outbred mice used for in vivo studies.

Despite the fact that there is a high burden of toxoplasmosis and transmission in Africa [13], there are no studies which have evaluated the immunopathology of Toxoplasma isolates from these countries. Further, there is little information available regarding the immune responses inherent to reactivated toxoplasmosis. Acute and chronic infections in the neurological model described above [24] was associated with increase in both IgM and IgG levels but following dexamethasone treatment, IgM levels declined but IgG levels continued on rising. The current study therefore sought to determine the profile of IFN-γ and IL-10, and organ pathology in immunocompetent and immunosuppressed mice infected with *T. gondii* isolated from a chicken in Kenya.

2. Materials and methods

2.1. Laboratory animals and ethical clearance

Prior to commencement of the study, all protocols and procedures used were reviewed and approved by the Institute of Primate Research, Institutional Animal Care and Use committee (Approval number: IRC/21/11). A total of 84 female BALB/c white mice were obtained from the rodent breeding facility Institute of Primate Research, Nairobi, Kenya. The mice were 6–8 weeks old and weighed 20–30 g. The mice were housed under standard laboratory conditions, in plastic cages (medium size cages; length 16.9 inches, width 10.5 inches, and height 5 inches) with wood shaving bedding and nesting material. Food (Mice Pellets®, Unga Feeds Ltd., Kenya), and drinking water were provided ad libitum.

2.2. *T. gondii* isolate and expansion

The *T. gondii* isolate used in this study was obtained from the brain of a free range chicken from Thika region, Kenya [26]. Briefly, the hen was sacrificed by cervical dislocation and the brain tissue collected under sterile conditions and processed for experimental infections. The brain was grounded and homogenized using tissue homogenizer. Enumeration of cysts was done as previously described [27], and the suspension was serially diluted with PBS (pH 7.2) to adjust to a desired final concentration of 15 tissue cysts/200 µl [24]. Three BALB/c mice were intraperitoneally injected each with 15 tissue cysts to allow for expansion of *T. gondii* cysts for use in experimental infection described below. The mice were monitored for 6 weeks post infection, euthanized using CO_2 and parasites isolated as stated earlier.

Prior to commencement of experimental work, the presence of *T. gondii* in the chicken samples was determined by extracting DNA from the brain sample using a Quick-gDNA™ MiniPrep Kit (Zymo research, USA) and nested PCR undertaken as previously described [13, 26]. Secondary amplification products were electrophoresed on 1.5% agarose gel stained with ethidium bromide and visualized under ultraviolet (UV) light.

2.3. Experimental design

The BALB/c mice were intraperitoneally infected with 15 *T. gondii* cysts in a 200 µl inoculum [24, 28]. In the first part of the experiment, 32 infected mice in groups of four were randomly chosen and euthanized by concentrated CO_2 inhalation on 3, 5 and 7 dpi for acute infection and 14, 21, 28, 35, 42 dpi for chronic infection. Sixteen BALB/C mice were controls and not infected with *T. gondii*.. After euthanasia, sampling for blood from the heart was done as previously described [23]. The liver, heart and spleen were also collected and preserved in 10% formalin and used for histology as described below.

At 42 dpi, 48 BALB/c mice previously infected with 15 cysts each, were divided into three groups of 16 mice each. The mice were treated with Dexamethasone (Decadron DexPak PHARMA Links, India) at dosages of 2.66 mg/kg (Group 1) and 5.32 mg/kg (Group 2) daily in drinking water over a period of 6 weeks [24, 29, 30]. Sixteen infected nontreated mice were used as controls (Group 3). Another 16 uninfected control mice were given untreated water (Group 4). The mice were monitored daily over 6 weeks for survival analysis and any clinical signs and mortalities were recorded. After every 2 weeks, four mice from each group were serially euthanized using concentrated carbon dioxide and sampling done as previously described above. Mice that showed any severe clinical signs of toxoplasmosis were anesthe-tized immediately using concentrated carbon dioxide and sampling of blood, done. The liver, heart and spleen were collected and preserved in 10% formalin.

2.4. IFN-γ and IL-10 levels

Serum for cytokine activities was prepared as previously described by Parasuraman *et al.* [31]. Cytokine production was evaluated using commercial ELISA kits according to the manufactur-er's instructions (MABTECH AB, Augustendalsvagen 19, Sweden). Briefly, each well of a 96-well high protein binding microtiter plate was coated with 100 µl/well of the respective monoclonal antibody diluted in PBS, pH 7.4 and incubated overnight at 4–8°C. The plates were washed twice with PBS (200 µl/well) and blocked by adding 200 µl/well of PBS with 0.05% Tween 20 containing 0.1% BSA (incubation buffer) and incubated for 1 hour at room temperature. Serum samples or recombinant mouse IFN-γ and IL-10 standards were then applied to the plates, and incubated for 2 h at 37°C. After washing, the respective biotinylated monoclonal antibody for IFN-γ and IL-10 was added and the plates incubated for an additional 1 h at 37°C. One hundred microliters of Streptavidin-ALP was then added to each microtiter well and incubated for 1 h at 37°C. After washing, 100 μl of p-nitrophenyl phosphate substrate was added to each well and the optical density measured at 405 nm for pNPP in an ELISA reader after suitable developing time. Cytokine concentrations were determined by reference to standard curves generated with murine recombinant cytokines. The sensitivity limits of the assays were 20 pg/ml for IL-10 and 4 pg/ml for IFN-γ as per the instructions of the manufacturer.

2.5. Histological analysis

Liver, spleen and heart were processed for paraffin embedding and sectioning. To determine the histological changes, tissue sections were stained with hematoxylin and eosin and observed under light microscope. The inflammation was assessed and scored histologically. The severity of the histopathological lesions in the heart was evaluated by grading the lesions using a modified random scale as previously described [32].

In the liver, the inflammatory lesions were quantified based on the degree of lymphocyte infiltration and hepatocyte necrosis as previously described [33]. Segments of spleen were scored for the enlargement of lymphocyte infiltrated areas and for the increased numbers of macrophages and necrotic cells previously described [34].

In these organs, the inflammatory changes were examined in two noncontinuous sections (40 μ distance between them) from each mouse in 25 microscopic fields using a 40× objective. The total inflammation score was determined from the summed scores of each mouse from each group or sampling time point and used for data analysis.

2.6. Data analysis

The results were entered into MS Excel program (Microsoft, USA) before being exported to GraphPad prism version 5.0 (GraphPad Software, USA) for statistical analysis. Statistical differences between the mice groups were determined by ANOVA; groups were considered statistically different if P ≤ 0.05.

3. Results

3.1. IFN-γ Levels

The mean of IFN-γ cytokine levels in the infected mice are as shown in **Figure 1**. There was a progressively significant (p < 0.001) increase in IFN-γ from 3.5 pg/ml (95%; CI: 2.93–4.07 at day 0 reaching 10.59 pg/ml, (95% CI: 9.03–12.15) at 35 dpi. The noninfected control group did not display any significant increase in IFN-γ cytokine levels and remained decreased at all time points compared to the infected group.

After treatment with dexamethasone, IFN-γ productions levels progressively declined at time points between 42 and 84 dpi. The decline in the 2.66 mg/kg/day of dexamethasone treated mice (Group 1) was from 17.84 pg/ml (95% CI: 1.60–34.08) at 42 dpi to 10.02 pg/ml (95% CI: 2.98–17.07) at 84 dpi (**Figure 2**).

The corresponding decline in the 2.66 mg/kg/day of dexamethasone treated mice (Group 2) was from 15.51 pg/ml (95% CI:–0.64–31.66) at 42 dpi to 7.89 pg/ml (95%; CI: 3.02–12.73.50) at

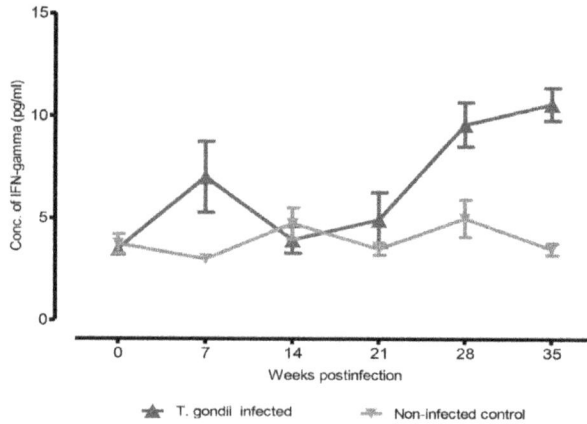

Figure 1. Levels of IFN-γ in serum of BALB/c infected with *T. gondii* during the early (7–14 dpi) and late stages (21–35 dpi) of infection. The data are expressed as the means ± SEM.

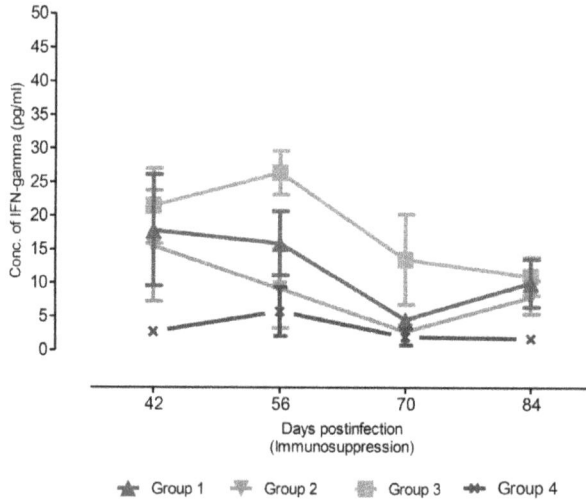

Figure 2. Mean levels of IFN-γ in serum in BALB/c infected with *T. gondii* and after dexamethasone treatment. The results are expressed as the means ± SEM of 4 mice. Group 1 = *T. gondii* infected dexamethasone treated (2.66 mg/kg/day); Group 2 = *T. gondii* infected dexamethasone treated (5.32 mg/kg/day); Group 3 = *T. gondii* infected; Group 4 = Noninfected control.

84 dpi. The decrease in IFN-γ levels was associated with increased dose, although the difference between the 2 doses were not significant (P > 0.05). The IFN-γ levels in the infected nontreated mice (Group 3) increased from 21.48 pg/ml (95%CI: 10.59–32.38) at 42 dpi to 26.38 pg/ml (95% CI: 20.01–32.75) at 56 dpi and thereafter, a progressive decline in IFN-γ levels reaching 13.53 pg/ml (95% CI: 0.42–26.64) and 11.03 pg/ml (95% CI: 5.43–16.64) at 70 and 84 dpi, respectively. Mice in the infected nontreated group (Group 3) maintained significantly (P < 0.001) increased levels of IFN-γ compared to the infected treated mice (**Figure 2**).

3.2. IL-10 levels

The levels of IL10 also increased following *T. gondii* infection. The levels significantly (P < 0.001) increased from 3.5 pg/ml (95%; CI: 2.93–4.07) at day 0 post-infection reaching 99.6 pg/ml (95% CI: 83.62–115.58) at 7 dpi and remained elevated up to day 35 dpi (119.6 pg/ml; 95%; CI: 106.27–124.45) (**Figure 3**).

Following dexamethasone treatment, the levels of IL-10 maintained a downward trend (**Figure 4**). In the mice treated with 2.66 mg/kg/day of DXM, the levels ranged between 135.66 pg/ml (95% CI: 82.79–188.54) at 42 dpi and dropped to 71.73 pg/ml (95% CI: 45.67–97.79) at 84 dpi. In the group treated with 5.32 mg/kg/day, the IL-10 level was 116.92 pg/ml (95% CI: 89.69–144.15) at 42 dpi and dropped to 55.59 pg/ml (95% CI: 40.77–70.43) at 84 dpi. The infected group (group 3) recorded a decreased IL-10 concentration ranging between 141.97 pg/ml (95% CI: 134.26–149.68) at 42 dpi and 99.71 pg/ml (95% CI: 77.16–122.27) at 84 dpi. Mice in the infected group recorded significantly (P < 0.01) elevated IL-10 levels compared to the treated groups at all time points.

3.3. Histological changes in the peripheral organs of BALB/c mice infected with *T. gondii*

In general, the histopathological changes in the liver, heart and spleen of infected mice consisted of mild-to-moderate congestion and detectable multifocal or focal inflammatory infiltrate. Between 3 and 14 dpi, the liver showed increased pathology characterized by hepatic necrosis, infiltration of lymphocytes and macrophages scattered in portal triad areas (**Figure 5**). The inflammatory scores increased from 1.2 (±0.49) at 3 dpi to 2.0 (±0.316) at 7 dpi. The highest inflammatory score was recorded at 14 dpi (2.8 ± 0.2) and thereafter, a progressive significant decline in inflammatory score (P < 0.001) at 42 dpi (1.4 ± 0.4) was observed.

Following dexamethasone treatment, the mice treated with 2.66 mg/kg/day (Group 1) and 5.32 mg/kg/day (Group 2) of dexamethasone showed varied degrees of inflammatory responses. For the mice treated with 2.66 mg/kg/day of dexamethasone, an inflammatory score of 1.4 (±0.245) and 2.0 (±0.00) was observed between 56 and 84 dpi, respectively, while the mice treated with 5.32 mg/kg/day (Group 2) of dexamethasone recorded an inflammatory score of 1.6 (±0.245) and 2.6 (±0.25) at 56 and 84 dpi, respectively. On the other hand, the infected nontreated mice presented an inflammatory score of 0.6 (±0.245) at 42 dpi but did not significantly (P > 0.05 change with the progression of the infection maintaining at 0.8 (±0.2) at 56, 70 and 84 dpi. Although the treated mice presented with progressively increased inflammatory scores there was no significant difference (P > 0.05) in the liver inflammatory response between the same groups.

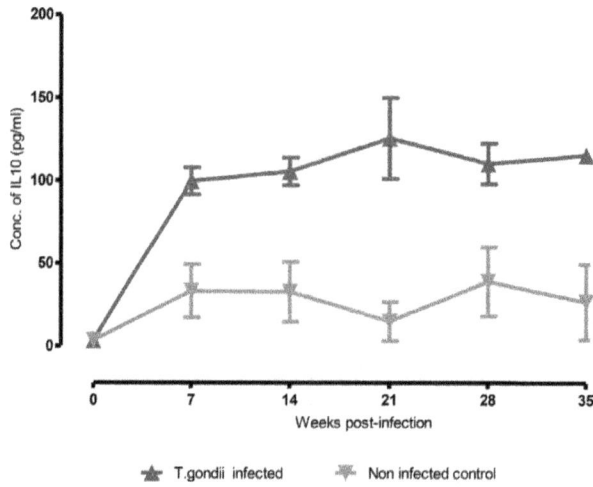

Figure 3. Mean levels of IL-10 in serum of BALB/c infected with *T. gondii* during the early (7–14 dpi) and late stages (21–35 dpi) of infection before treatment. The data are expressed as the means ± SEM.

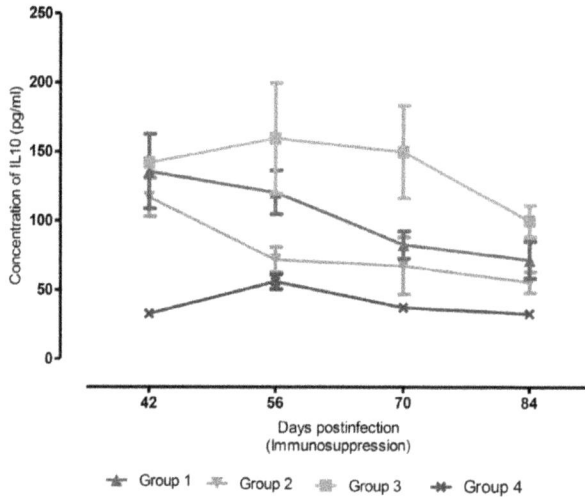

Figure 4. Levels of IL-10 in serum from BALB/c mice infected with *T. gondii* and after dexamethasone treatment. The data are expressed as the means ± SEM of 4 mice. Group 1 = *T. gondii* infected dexamethasone treated (2.66 mg/kg/day); Group 2 = *T. gondii* infected dexamethasone treated (5.32 mg/kg/day); Group 3 = *T. gondii* infected; Group 4 = Noninfected mice.

In the heart of infected mice, the histopathological lesions were relatively fewer compared to those in liver and were characterized by inflammatory infiltrates (**Figure 6**). The inflammatory score at 7 dpi was 1.75 (±0.25) and this was followed by a significant (P < 0.001) decrease reaching the lowest inflammatory score of 1.25 (±0.25) at 35 dpi. However, treatment with dexamethasone markedly increased the severity and number of myocardial lesions in these infected animals. The toxoplasma infected group (Group 3) presented with

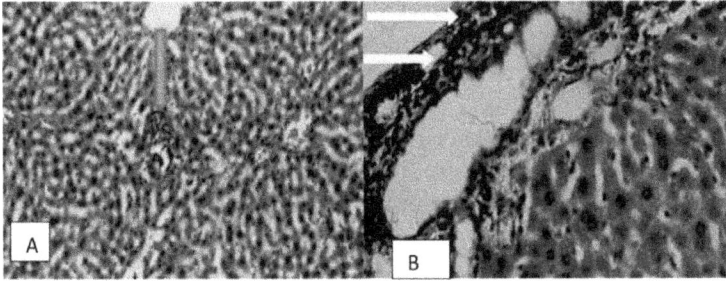

Figure 5. Liver of infected and treated mice showing dense granulomas, irregularly distributed (arrows) (A) and infiltrations of inflammatory cells (arrows) at the portal triad (B).

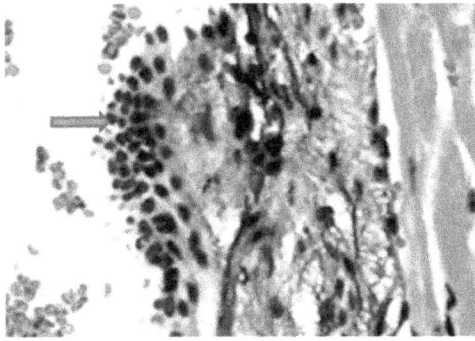

Figure 6. Heart of BALB/c mice showing inflammatory cell infiltrations (arrow).

higher inflammatory lesions at the time of treatment (day 42 dpi; P < 0.01). However, at 56, 70 and 84 dpi, an increasing inflammatory score was noted although there was no significant difference (P > 0.05). All the heart tissues of mice from group 1 recorded an inflammatory score of 1.25 (±0.25) at 56, 70 and 84 dpi (P > 0.05) while group 2 recorded a significant (p < 0.01) inflammatory score of 1.25 (±0.25); 1.5 (±0.289) and 2.5 (±0.289) at 56, 70 and 84 dpi, respectively. The uninfected control group (Groups 4) did not show any myocardial lesions at all time points.

The spleen was also affected by *T. gondii* but unlike the liver, the inflammatory response started from 5 dpi. The infected mice spleens from the infected treated mice presented general disorganization of the germinal centers at 70 dpi. The marginal zone disappeared and the limits between the disorganized germinal center and the red pulp were blurred. The noninfected mice spleens exhibited no change in the organizational of the germinal centers.

4. Discussion

In the present study, BALB/c mice infected with *T. gondii* showed that IFN-γ productions were markedly increased after *T. gondii* infection. This observation is consistent with a previous study in mice by Gazzinelli *et al.* [35], where equally, IFN-γ levels were exceedingly elevated at the disease onset. Once released, IFNγ binds to the IFNγ receptor (IFN-γR), which eventually leads to the activation of IFN-γ signals "signal transducer and activator of transcription 1" (STAT1); [36]. These factors acts on macrophages and monocytes inducing the transcription of various genes involved in anti-parasitic responses including production of toxic reactive-oxygen species [37, 38]. The high levels of IFN-γ production levels are suggestive of its early involvement in parasite clearance [39]. The secretion of IFN-γ increases the phagocyte activity of macrophages and also triggers the conversion of tachyzoites into bradyzoites leading to chronicity [40, 41, 42]. The cytokine also prevents bradyzoite rupture, allowing long specific protection against new parasite infections and is hence responsible for regulation of *T. gondii* load and distribution in the tissues [43]. Although IFN-γ-dependent pro - inflammatory cytokines are essential for resistance to *T. gondii* infection, an over-production of inflammatory cytokine, IFN-γ can result in serious tissue damage [38] . Therefore, the intensity of the immune responses mounted against *T. gondii* just like any other infection must be regulated to avoid exaggerated immune-pathologic effects due to excessive inflammation.

In the current study, the IFN-γ levels were significantly depressed in the dexamethasone-treated *T. gondii* infected mice [44].). Dexamethasone administration have been shown to induce programmed cell death in developing lymphocytes. Harold *et al.* [45] has shown that dexamethasone is a potent suppressor of cytokine production in T cells. This drug, just like other glucocorticoids, act by binding to the glucocorticoid receptor, which blocks the expression of pro-inflammatory cytokines and adhesion molecules. Previous early studies done by Hunter *et al.* [20] showed that mice lacking T cells do not survive latent infection while depletion in T cells during the chronic phase or as a result of immunosuppression re-activates the disease [35].

In the current study, the IL-10 levels were also elevated during the acute and chronic infection and there was also a decline in immunosuppressed mice (42–84 dpi). This anti-inflammatory cytokine, has the ability to antagonize T helper 1 (Th1) responses [46]. IL-10 is considered to be an inhibitor of Th1 and Th2 immune responses [47, 48, 49]. Therefore, the role of IL-10 cytokines secreted by macrophages, monocytes, B cells, and CD4+ and CD8+ T cells during both the acute and the chronic phases of infection in both immunocompetent and immunosuppressed mice is to acts broadly on accessory cells and adaptive cells responses to downregulate or limit the consequences of an exaggerated inflammatory response and major histocompatibility complex and costimulatory molecule expression [20, 47, 50, 51]. This cytokine also prevents tissue immune destruction through immunomodulation [18] and has been identified as a factor induced by *T. gondii* infection [35, 52] that can contribute to the suppression of T cell function [53, 54].

Toxoplasma gondii infection caused different pathological manifestations as shown in this study. In the early infection, BALB/c mice displayed intense inflammatory lesions in the liver, heart as well as disorganization of the germinal centers of the spleen, suggesting a strong immune response in the pathogenesis of the disease. In the spleen, the white pulp appeared enlarged due to cellular proliferation and its limit with the red pulp started to disappear.

The detectable changes in the splenic architecture of the structures in the spleen of dexamethasone treated mice have been associated with a decreased ability to mount an immune response against the toxoplasma parasites [55]. Multiple mechanisms have been implicated in splenic disorganization, including CD8+ T cell-mediated cytolysis of infected stromal cells or follicular dendritic cells and marginal-zone macrophages [56].

The results of the present study showed that chronically infected nontreated mice had an increase in mononuclear cells organ infiltrations upon infection. The recruitment of inflammatory cells as was the case in these organs, is one of the most important immune mechanisms induced by IFN-γ and is geared towards control of parasite multiplication. These cells could also be responsible for the higher levels of cytokines observed in the initial stage of *T. gondii* infection observed in the study. However, although there was a decline in the cytokine levels in the immunosuppressed mice, there was marked infiltration of mononuclear cells in the organs, resulting in myocarditis and hepatitis. This could be a reflection of reactivation and spread of toxoplasma parasites following decline in inflammatory response hindering the control and proliferation of the parasite [57].

5. Conclusions

The results of this study indicates that immunological and pathological features of *T. gondii* in immunosuppressed BALB/c mice mimic toxoplasmosis in immunosuppressed humans as it occurs during advanced HIV infection when CD4+ counts are low. The infection in immunocompetent host was associated with elevated IFN-γ and IL-10 which declined after immunosuppression. However, in both competent and immunocompetent mice, the pathological signs evident in the study were myocarditis, hepatitis characterized by mononuclear cell infiltration. Splenic exhaustion characterized by loss of normal spleen architecture also characterized the infection.

Acknowledgements

This work was funded by Jomo Kenyatta University of Agriculture and Technology (JKUAT)-Research production and Extension. The authors are grateful to the technical assistance provided by IPR staff including Samson Mutura, Tom Adino, Esther Kagasi and Caroline Jerono.

Competing interests

The authors declare that they have no financial or personal relationship(s) that may have inappropriately influenced them in writing this book chapter.

Author details

John Mokua Mose[1,2], David Muchina Kamau[2], John Maina Kagira[3*], Naomi Maina[4], Maina Ngotho[5], Lucy Mutharia[6] and Simon Muturi Karanja[2]

*Address all correspondence to: jkagira@gmail.com

1 Department of Medical Laboratory Science, School of Medicine and Health Sciences, Kenya Methodist University, Nairobi, Kenya

2 Department of Public Health, Jomo Kenyatta University of Agriculture and Technology (JKUAT), Nairobi, Kenya

3 Department of Animal Sciences, Jomo Kenyatta University of Agriculture and Technology (JKUAT), Nairobi, Kenya

4 Department of Biochemistry, Jomo Kenyatta University of Agriculture and Technology (JKUAT), Nairobi, Kenya

5 Department of Animal Health and Production, Mount Kenya University, Thika, Kenya

6 Department of Molecular and Cellular Biology, Guelph University, Guelph, ON, Canada

References

[1] Dubey JP, Beattie CP. Toxoplasmosis of Animals and Man. Boca Raton, Fla, USA: CRC Press; 1988

[2] Hill D, Dubey JP. *Toxoplasma gondii*: Transmission, diagnosis and prevention. Clinical Microbiology and Infection. 2002;8(10):634-640

[3] Mas Bakal P, Khan AA, Goedbloed E. Toxoplasmosis in Kenya-A pilot study. East African Medical Journal. 1968;45:557-562

[4] Bowry TR, Camargo ME, Kinyanjui M. Sero-epidemiology of *Toxoplasma gondii* infection in young children in Nairobi, Kenya. Transactions of the Royal Society of Tropical Medicine and Hygiene. 1986;80:439-441

[5] Griffin L, Williams KA. Serological and parasitological survey of blood donors in Kenya for toxoplasmosis. Transactions of the Royal Society of Tropical Medicine and Hygiene. 1983;77:763-766

[6] Brindle R, Holliman R, Gilks C, Waiyaki P. Toxoplasma antibodies in HIV-positive patients from Nairobi. Transactions of the Royal Society of Tropical Medicine and Hygiene. 1991;85:750-751

[7] Lodenyo H, Sitati SM, Rogena E. Case report: Reactivated toxoplasmosis presenting with non-tender hepatomegaly in a patient with HIV infection. AJHS. 2007;14:97-98

[8] Jowi JO, Mativo PM, Musoke SS. Clinical and laboratory characteristics of hospitalised patients with neurological manifestations of HIV/AIDS at the Nairobi hospital. East African Medizinhistorisches Journal. 2007;**84**:67-76

[9] Wiseman RA, Fleck DG, Woodruff AW. Toxoplasmal and toxocaral infections: A clinical investigation into their relationship. British Medical Journal. 1970;**4**:152-153

[10] Chunge RN, Desai M, Simwa JM, Omondi BE, Kinoti SN. Prevalence of antibodies to *Toxoplasma gondii* in serum samples from pregnant women and cord blood at Kenyatta National Hospital, Nairobi. The East African Medical Journal. 1989;**66**:560

[11] Kalter SS, Kagan IG, Kuntz RE. Antibodies to parasities in Kenya baboons: Papio sp. Transactions of the Royal Society of Tropical Medicine and Hygiene. 1969;**63**:684-686

[12] Njuguna AN, Kagira JM, Karanja SM, Nnotho M, Mutharia L, Naomi WM. Prevalence of *Toxoplasma gondii* and other gastrointestinal parasites in domestic cats from households in Thika Region, Kenya. BioMed Research International. 2017;**2017**:6. Article ID: 7615810

[13] Thiong'o SK, Ichagichu JM, Ngotho M, Aboge GO, Kagira JM, Karanja SM, Maina NN. Use of the nested polymerase chain reaction for detection of *Toxoplasma gondii* in slaughterhouse workers in Thika District, Kenya. South African Medical Journal. 2016;**106**(4):417-419

[14] Dubey JP, Karhemere S, Dahl E, Sreekumar C, Diabate A. First biologic and genetic characterization of *Toxoplasma gondii* isolates from chickens from Africa (Democratic Republic of Congo, Mali, Burkina Faso, and Kenya). Journal of Parasitology. 2005;**91**: 69-72. DOI: 10.1645/GE-410R

[15] Velmurugan GV, Dubey JP, Su C. Genotyping studies of *Toxoplasma gondii* isolates from Africa revealed that the archetypal clonal lineages predominate as in North America and Europe. Veterinary Parasitology. 2008;**155**:314-318. DOI: 10.1016/j.vetpar.2008.04.021

[16] Tenter AM, Anja RH, Louis MW. *Toxoplasma gondii*: From animals to humans. International Journal for Parasitology. 2000;**30**:1217-1258

[17] Denkers EY, Gazzinelli RT. Regulation of function of T-cell-mediated immunity during *Toxoplasma gondii* infection. Clinical Microbiology Reviews. 1998;**11**(4):569-588

[18] Gaddi PJ, Yap GS. Cytokine regulation of immunopathology in toxoplasmosis. Immunology and Cell Biology. 2007;**85**(2):155-159

[19] Lindberg RE, Frenkel JK. Cellular immunity to toxoplasma and besnoitia in hamsters: Specificity and the effects of cortisol. Infection and Immunity. 1977;**15**(3):855-862

[20] Hunter C, Subauste C, Remington J. The role of cytokines in toxoplasmosis. Biotherapy. 1994;**7**(3):237-247

[21] Brinkmann V, Remington JS, Sharma SD. Vaccination of mice with the protective F3G3 antigen of *Toxoplasma gondii* activates CD4+ but not CD8+ T cells and induces Toxoplasma specific IgG antibody. Molecular Immunology. 1993;**30**(4):353-358

[22] Vossenkamper A, Struck D, Esquivel CA, Went T, Takeda K, Akira S, Pfeffer K, Alber G, Lochner M, Forster I, Liesenfeld O. Both IL-12 and IL-18 contribute to small intestinal Th1-type immunopathology following oral infection with *Toxoplasma gondii*, but IL-12 is dominant over IL-18 in parasite control. European Journal of Immunology. 2004;**34**(11):3197-3207

[23] Liesenfeld O. Immune responses to *Toxoplasma gondii* in the gut. Immunobiology. 1999; **201**(2):229-239

[24] Mose JM, Kamau DM, Kagira JM, Maina M, Ngotho M, Njuguna A, Karanja SM. Development of neurological mouse model for toxoplasmosis using *Toxoplasma gondii* isolated from chicken in Kenya. Pathology Research International. 2017;**2017**:8

[25] Falangola MF, Reichler BS, Petito CK. Histopathology of cerebral toxoplasmosis in human immunodeficiency virus infection: A comparison between patients with early-onset and late-onset acquired immunodeficiency syndrome. Journal of Human Pathology. 1994;**25**(10):1091-1109

[26] Mose JM, Kagira JM, Karanja SM, Ngotho M, Kamau DM, Njuguna AN, NW, Maina NW. Detection of natural *Toxoplasma gondii* infection in chicken in Thika Region of Kenya using nested polymerase chain reaction. BioMed Research International. 2016;**2016**:5. Article ID: 7589278

[27] Ole A. OIE manual of diagnostic tests and vaccines for terrestrial animals. Toxoplasmosis. 2008;**1**(6):1286

[28] Weiss LM, Kim K. The development and biology of bradyzoites of *Toxoplasma gondii*. Frontiers in Bioscience: A Journal and Virtual Library. 2000;**5**:D391-D405

[29] Kawedia JD, Janke L, Funk AJ, Ramsey LB, Liu C, Jenkins D, Boyd KL, Relling MV. Substrain-specific differences in survival and osteonecrosis incidence in a mouse model. Comparative Medicine. 2012;**62**(6):466-471

[30] Nicoll S, Wright SW, Maley SB, Buxton D. A mouse model of recrudescence of *Toxoplasma gondii* infection. Journal of Medical Microbiology. 1997;**46**:263-266

[31] Parasuraman S, Raveendran R, Kesavan R. Blood sample collection in small laboratory animals. Journal of Pharmacology and Pharmacotherapeutics. 2010;**1**(2):87-93

[32] Dong R, Liu P, Wee L, Butany J, Sole MJ. Verapamil ameliorates the clinical and pathological course of murine myocarditis. Journal of Clinical Investigation. 1992;**90**(5):2022-2030

[33] Ishak K, Baptista A, Bianchi L, Callea F, De Groote J, Gudat F, Denk H, Desmet V, Korb G, MacSween RN. Histologic grading and staging of chronic hepatitis. Journal of Hepatology. 1995;**22**(6):696-699

[34] Evangelos J, Bourboulis G, Tziortzioti V, Koutoukas P, Baziaka F, Raftogiannis M, Antonopoulou A, Adamis T, Sabracos L, Giamarellou H. Clarithromycin is an effective immunomodulator in experimental pyelonephritis caused by pan-resistant *Klebsiella pneumoniae*. Journal of Antimicrobial Chemotherapy. 2006;**57**(5):937-944

[35] Gazzinelli RT, Hartley JW, Fredrickson TN, Chattopadhyay SK, Sher A, Morse HC. Opportunistic infections and retrovirus-induced immunodeficiency: Studies of acute and chronic infections with *Toxoplasma gondii* in mice infected with LP-BM5 murine leukemia viruses. Infection and Immunity. 1992;**60**(10):4394-4401

[36] Kim SK, Karasov A, Boothroyd JC. Bradyzoite-specific surface antigen SRS9 plays a role in maintaining *Toxoplasma gondii* persistence in the brain and in host control of parasite replication in the intestine. Infection and Immunity. 2007;**75**:1626-1634

[37] Arsenijevic D, Bilbao FD, Giannakopoulos P, Girardier L, Samec S, Richard D. A role for interferon-gamma in the hypermetabolic response to murine toxoplasmosis. European Cytokine Network. 2001;**12**:518-527

[38] Mordue DG, Monroy F, La Regina M, Dinarello CA, Sibley LD. Acute toxoplasmosis leads to lethal overproduction of Th1 cytokines. Journal of Immunology. 2001;**167**:4574-4584

[39] Lee YH, Noh HJ, Hwang OS, Lee SK, Shin DW. Seroepidemiological study of *Toxoplasma gondii* infection in the rural area Okcheon-gun, Korea. Korean Journal of Parasitology. 2000;**38**(4):251-256

[40] Bohne W, Heesemann J, Gross U. Induction of bradyzoite specific *Toxoplasma gondii* antigens in gamma interferon treated mouse macrophages. Infection and Immunity. 1993;**61**(3):1141-1145

[41] Ely KH, Kasper LH, Khan IA. Augmentation of the CD8+ T cell response by IFN-gamma in IL-12-deficient mice during *Toxoplasma gondii* infection. Journal of Immunology. 1999;**162**(9):5449-5554

[42] Nijhawan R, Bansal R, Gupta N, Beke N, Kulkarni P, Gupta A. Intraocular cysts of *Toxoplasma gondii* in patients with necrotizing retinitis following periocular/intraocular triamcinolone injection. Ocular Immunology and Inflammation. 2013;**21**(5):396-399

[43] Capron A, Dessaint JP. Vaccination against parasitic diseases: Some alternative concepts for the definition of protective antigens. Annales de l'Institut Pasteur. Immunologie. 1988;**139**:109-117

[44] Gazzinelli RT, Wysocka M, Hayashi S, Denkers EY, Hieny S, Caspar P, Trinchieri G, Sher A. Parasite-induced IL-12 stimulates early IFN-γ synthesis and resistance during acute infection with *Toxoplasma gondii*. Journal of Immunology. 1994;**153**(6):2533-2543

[45] Herold MJ, McPherson KG, Reichardt HM. Glucocorticoids in T cell apoptosis and function. Cellular and Molecular Life Sciences. 2006;**63**(1):60-72

[46] Fiorentino DF, Zlotnik A, Vieira P, Mosmann TR, Howard M, Moore KW, A O'Garra AO. IL-10 acts on the antigen-presenting cell to inhibit cytokine production by Th1 cells. The Journal of Immunology. 1991;**146**(10):3444-3451

[47] Moore KW, de Waal Malefyt R, Coffman RL, O'Garra A. Interleukin-10 and the interleukin-10 receptor. Annual Review and Immunology. 2001;**19**:683-765

[48] Lieberman LA, Hunter CA. The role of cytokines and their signaling pathways in the regulation of immunity to *Toxoplasma gondii*. International Reviews of Immunology. 2002;**21**(4-5):373-403

[49] O'Garra A, Vieira P. T(H)1 cells control themselves by producing interleukin-10. Nature Reviews. Immunology. 2007;**7**(6):425-428

[50] Hall AO, Beiting DP, Tato C, John B, Oldenhove G, Lombana CG, Pritchard GH, Silver JS, Bouladoux N, Stumhofer JS. The cytokines interleukin 27 and interferon-γ promote distinct Treg cell populations required to limit infection-induced pathology. Immunity. 2012;**37**:511-523

[51] Gerard EK, Jay CH, Kenneth WB, Philip MH. Immunological decision-making: How does the immune system decide to mount a helper T-cell response? Immunology. 2008;**123**(3):326-338

[52] Burke JM, Roberts CW, Hunter CA, Murray M, Alexander J. Temporal differences in the expression of mRNA for IL-10 and IFN-γ in the brains and spleens of C57BL/10 mice infected with *Toxoplasma gondii*. Parasite Immunology. 1994;**16**:305-314

[53] Candolfi E, Hunter CA, Remington JS. Roles of γ interferon and other cytokines in suppression of the spleen cell proliferative response to concavalin A and Toxoplasma antigens during actue toxoplasmosis. Infection and Immunity. 1995;**63**:751-756

[54] Khan IA, Matsuura T, Kasper LH. IL-10 mediates immunosuppression following primary infection with *Toxoplasma gondii* in mice. Parasite Immunology. 1995;**17**:185-195

[55] Odermatt B, Eppler M, Leist TP, Hengartner H, Zinkernagel RM. Virus-triggered acquired immunodeficiency by cytotoxic T-cell dependent destruction of antigen-presenting cells and lymph follicle structure. National Academy of Sciences of the United States. 1991;**88**(18):8252-8256

[56] Mueller SN, Matloubian M, Clemens DM, Sharpe AH, Freeman GJ, Gangappa S, Larsen CP, Ahmed A. Viral targeting of fibroblastic reticular cells contributes to immunosuppression and persistence during chronic infection. Proceedings of the National Academy of Sciences. 2007;**104**(39):15430-15435

[57] Kaplan JE, Benson C, Holmes KH, Brooks JT, Pau A, Masur H. Guidelines for prevention and treatment of opportunistic infections in HIV-infected adults and adolescents: Recommendations from CDC, the National Institutes of Health, and the HIV Medicine Association of the Infectious Diseases Society of America. MMWR Recommendations and Reports. 2009;**58**(RR04):1-198

Malaria Pathophysiology as a Syndrome: Focus on Glucose Homeostasis in Severe Malaria and Phytotherapeutics Management of the Disease

Greanious Alfred Mavondo, Joy Mavondo,
Wisdom Peresuh, Mary Dlodlo and Obadiah Moyo

Additional information is available at the end of the chapter

http://dx.doi.org/10.5772/intechopen.79698

Abstract

Severe malaria presents with varied pathophysiological manifestations to include derangement in glucose homeostasis. The changes in glucose management by the infected human host emanate from both *Plasmodium* parasitic and host factors and/or influences which are aimed at creating a proliferative advantage to the parasite. This also includes morphological changes that that take place to both infected and uninfected cells as structural alterations occur on the cell membranes to allow for increased nutrients (glucose) transportation into the cells. Without the availability, effective and efficient intervention there is a high cost incurred by the human host. Hyperglycaemia, hypoglycaemia and hyperinsulinemia are critical aspects displayed in severe malaria. Conventional treatment to malaria renders itself hostile to the host with negative glucose metabolism changes experiences in the young, pregnant women and malaria naïve individuals. In malaria, therefore, host effects, parasite imperatives and treatment regimens play a pivotal role in the return to wellness of the patient. Phytotherapeutics are emerging as treatment alternatives that ameliorate glucose homeostasis alternations as well as combat malaria parasitaemia. The phytochemicals e.g. triterpenes, have been shown to alleviate the "disease" and "parasitic" aspects of malaria pointing at key aspects in ameliorating malaria glucose homeostasis fallings-out that are experienced in malaria.

Keywords: malaria, glucose homeostasis, hypoglycaemia, hyperglycaemia, GLUT1, GLUT4, HfHT, hyperinsulinemia, phytochemicals, asiatic acid, triterpenes

1. Introduction

Malaria is one of the most prevalent parasitic diseases ever to infect the human being with causalities exceeding 200 million a year of mostly children <5 years of age, pregnant women, and people form none-endemic areas who happen to be non-immune to the disease [1]. Continuous and frequent infections for the Plasmodium parasites from holoendemic areas induces immune semi-protection to the malaria disease mostly the malaria naïve visitors [2]. There are several parasites species of the *Plasmodium genus* (>100 species) but only a few have the correct virulence to cause malaria in humans. These include *Plasmodium falciparum*, *Plasmodium vivax*, *Plasmodium ovale*, *Plasmodium malariae* and the zoonotic *Plasmodium knowlesi*. These parasites give diverse malarial syndromes with *P. falciparum* giving the most virulent and fatal disease. Even with this infection, the disease poses varying degrees of severity with one extreme displaying an asymptomatic blood smear erythrocytic phase positive infection and the other extreme displaying severe malarial disease with high mortality risk [3]. Severe malaria (SM) manifests as clinical and pathological heterogeneous complications that differ in the rate of occurrence, age of the subjects and geographical distributions [4] following disease patterns and time course that may be predictable or completely obscure to researchers, clinicians and the subjects alike.

While cerebral malaria (CM) ranks as the most dangerous, with the highest fatality of all forms of SM, severe malaria anaemia (SMA) [5] follows a close second in sub-Saharan Africa. Hypoglycaemia [6–8], hypotension, acute kidney injury (AKI) [9], acute respiratory distress syndrome (ARDS) and acute lung injury (ALI) [10], pulmonary oedema, non-respiratory acidosis (nRD) and hyperlactaemia [11–13], bleeding and blood clotting irregularities with thrombocytopaenia, aberrant inflammatory response [14] and pre-hepatic jaundice are often presented in SM although at varying incidence and prevalence [15]. The pathophysiology and parasitic influences are indeed variable in individuals. However, in all complications there is a base line of metabolic and homeostatic dysfunctions that have been observed over time, especially of glucose and associated processes that seem to be ameliorated by agents trained at the "disease" aspect of malaria [8, 10, 16] as compared to the "parasitic" influences.

Several factors tend to influence glucose homeostasis in malarial infections. These include parasite metabolism, malarial pyrexia, human host hormonal changes, inflammatory soluble mediators (cytokines and chemokines), natural immunological responses irregularities, malarial anorexia and cachexic tendencies and gastrointestinal disturbances [11]. There is a general trend observed in the glucose homeostasis that follows a tendency towards hypoglycaemic phenotype which, without appropriate intervention, evolves into end stage disease hyperglycaemia. Insufficient hormonal effectiveness associated with immunological-inflammatory aberrations of severe malaria play a pivotal role in the malaria-induced glucose homeostasis decline.

Insulin is the foremost and most important hormone that is involved in the plasma glucose homeostasis and is counter regulated by almost other hormones that are involved in carbohydrate metabolism such as glucagon, thyroid hormones (thyroxine and triiodothyronine) growth hormone, cortisol, somatomedins, somatostatins, gastrointestinal secretin of the other hormones.

In malaria, the intracellular-erythrocytic malaria parasite partly influences glucose homeostasis. Generally, the red blood cell (RBC) or erythrocyte is categorised as an insulin-independent tissue having no plasma membrane insulin receptors (IR's). Glucose uptake by the RBC's is transported across their plasma membrane through the facilitation of glucose transporter 1 (GLUT 1). There is a significant and dramatic transformation of parasitized RBC's (pRBC's) plasma membranes after invasion by the *Plasmodium* parasite through insertion of various transmembrane proteins forming knobs which are interactions between the host and parasite proteins. These structures are formed from pRBC proteins such as spectrin and actin combining with parasite derived molecules such as ring-infected erythrocyte surface antigen (RESA), knob associated histidine-rich protein (KAHRP), mature parasite-infected erythrocyte surface antigen (MESA), *Plasmodium falciparum* erythrocyte membrane protein 1 (PfEMP1) and PfEMP3 [17]. These protein remodel the pRBC for increase parasite virulence, expedite the movement of parasite requirements into and discarded products out of the pRBC to meet the needs of the growing intra-erythrocytic food vacuole enclosed parasites [18]. There is a distinct change that occurs in the cell membrane structure and function in pRBC's with targeted disruption parasite proteins genes invariably leading to changes in membrane rigidity and, cytoadherence and glucose transportation [19, 20] (**Figure 1**). The resultant changes in the cell membrane is necessary to maintain the structural formation or remodelling necessary for exchanges between the food vacuole and the host cell cytoplasm. Channels formed in the plasma membrane need to be maintained without disruption until the parasite intra-erythrocyte parasite has matured. This also means the mechanism for glucose transport into the pRBC's are also maintained.

The main parasitic energy source is glucose. The *P. falciparum* hexose transporter (*Pf*HT), which transports both glucose and fructose, is the main transporter of glucose shuttle from the cytoplasm to the parasitophorous vacuole [15, 21–23]. Within the parasite vacuole, glucose concentration may be higher than that in the pRBC due to the efficient transport of the *Pf*HT driving hypoglycaemia to some extent, although it was thought to be an passive action before [24].

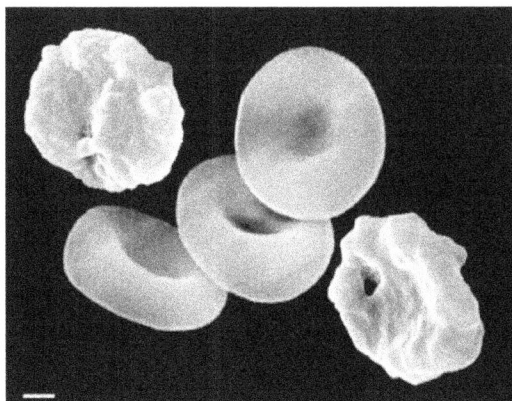

Figure 1. Scanning electron micrograph of normal RBC and *Plasmodium falciparum* pRBC. The three normal RBC at the centre appear regular and smooth and have a biconcave structure. In contrast the two peripheral pRBC have an irregular and rough surface and have lost the biconcave structure. (Published with permission, Professor David Ferguson, Oxford University, Oxford, UK). Scale bar = 1 μm.

Also, pRBC anchor protein glycosylphosphatidylinositol (GPI) have an insulinomemetic effect that may also drive hypoglycaemia. However, insulin resistance seen in end-stage SM, fuels hyperglycaemia where insulin-dependent tissues like muscle and adipose tissue may be deficient of glucose intracellularly in the face of hyperinsulinism depicting glucose disturbances during SM [25]. Counter regulatory glucose metabolism also has been shown to increase gluconeogenesis in SM without necessarily increasing their activities due to the tissue resistance to insulin [26]. In addition to hormonal effects, inflammatory mediators play a crucial role in the hyperglycaemia experienced in SM.

It is imperative to explain the normal glucose homeostasis before a description of the pathophysiology of malarial glucose metabolism may be attempted. Here the process by which aberrant glucose metabolism occurs in SM is explored with critical emphasis on how management of the malaria disease may be useful in averting glucose homeostasis derangements.

1.1. Glucose homeostasis

Human blood glucose concentration control is one of the most tightly and acutely physiological processes. Glucose utilisation, storage and remarshalling takes place in diverse number of tissues to include in the blood. When carbohydrates are consumed, blood glucose diminishes in concentration through an insulin-stimulated glucose transport process into the skeletal muscles and adipose tissue for storage. Glucose is stored as glycogen in the skeletal muscles which is subsequently oxidised to provide energy following an active transport process.

Glucose transporter 4 (GLUT4) is the key player in modifiable whole-body glucose homeostasis and balance. Even after a huge caloric intake, elevated glucose concentrations are promptly restored to concentrations between 5 and 6 mmol/L which would vary to slightly lower concentration in times of long term starvation or considerable food intake deprivation. This way, severe dysfunctions induced by hypoglycaemia such as loss of consciousness and peripheral tissue noxiousness of chronic diabetes mellitus are forfended. In malaria, however, GLUT1 is more prominent in glucose transport in both the pRBC and the hepatocyte although GLUT2 is the resident transporter of glucose in the liver cells.

2. Glucose transporter 4 (GLUT4)

To modulate the glucose homeostasis, an exogenous glucose load transport into skeletal muscles is mediated by the solute carrier 2A4 (SLC2A4) gene coded protein GLUT4 which is a 12-transmembrane domains containing sugar transporter. GLUT4 is one of the 13 sugar transporter proteins (GLUT1-GLUT12 and HMIT) which are encoded in the human genome [27] which catalyse hexose transport across cell membranes through ATP-independent, facilitative diffusion mechanism [28].

There is a varied display of kinetics and substrate specificities amongst the sugar transporters with GLUT5 and GLUT11 specialising in the transport of fructose. There is a high expression of GLUT4 in adipose tissue and skeletal muscle although a selective cohort of other transporters are also present with GLUT1, GLUT5 and GLUT12 significantly contribute to the glucose uptake by muscle tissue [30, 31] while GLUT8, GLUT12, HMIT are also expressed by adipose tissue [27, 32]. GLUT4 remains in the cytoplasm when it is in its inactivated state making a unique and characteristic rapid response when plasma glucose concentrations are increased with an acute redistribution to the plasma membrane under the influence of insulin [33]. The cytoplasmic domains of GLUT4 provides the distinctive plasma membrane mobilizations capabilities of this sugar transporter in that it contains a unique sequence in its N- and COOH terminals (**Figure 2**). In the N-terminal GLUT4 has a critical phenylalanine residue [34], a dileucine and acidic motifs in the COOH terminus, which motifs directs kinetic facets of endocytosis and exocytosis recycling trafficking coordination [35, 36]. GLUT4 plays a critical role in both insulin signalling and plasma membrane trafficking [37].

Stimulation of GLUT4 recruitment to the surface of plasma membranes of muscle and adipose cells is carried out by insulin and exercise in a non-transcription or translation dependent process [38, 39]. However, the signalling mechanisms that are initiated by these two physiological stimulations leading to the translocation of GLUT4 and the uptake of glucose are distinct and separate [40, 41] as shown by the diagrammatic representation in **Figure 3**. This has a profound implication on the hyper-muscular/physical activities (physical movement or malaria pyrexia) and hyperinsulinemia that tend to be associated with malaria which may lead to and or worsen hypoglycaemia of malaria.

In the canonical insulin signalling pathway, activation of the insulin receptor (IR) tyrosine kinase triggers the process leading to insulin receptor substrate proteins (IRS) tyrosine phosphorylation and their recruitment of PI 3-kinase. PI 3-kinase catalyses the conversion of phosphatidylinositol (4,5)P2 to phosphatidylinositol (3,4,5)P3 (PIP3), which triggers protein kinase Akt activation through intermediate proteins PDK1 and Rictor/mTOR [42, 43].

A number of cellular stress signals enhance glucose uptake by skeletal muscle. Free fatty acids (FFT's), increased cytokines, endothelial reticulum stress, hypoxia, oxidative stress,

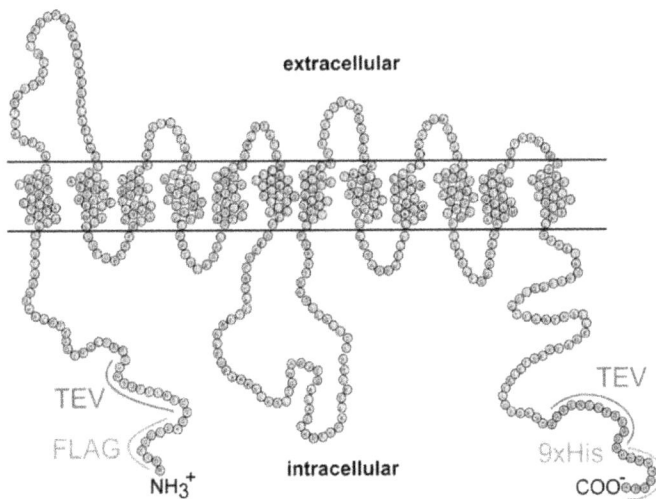

Figure 2. Predicted topology map of GLUT4. The membrane topology was predicted using the TOPCONS web server for consensus prediction of membrane protein topology and signal peptides [29]. Grey amino acids were added for aiding purification and removal of purification tags.

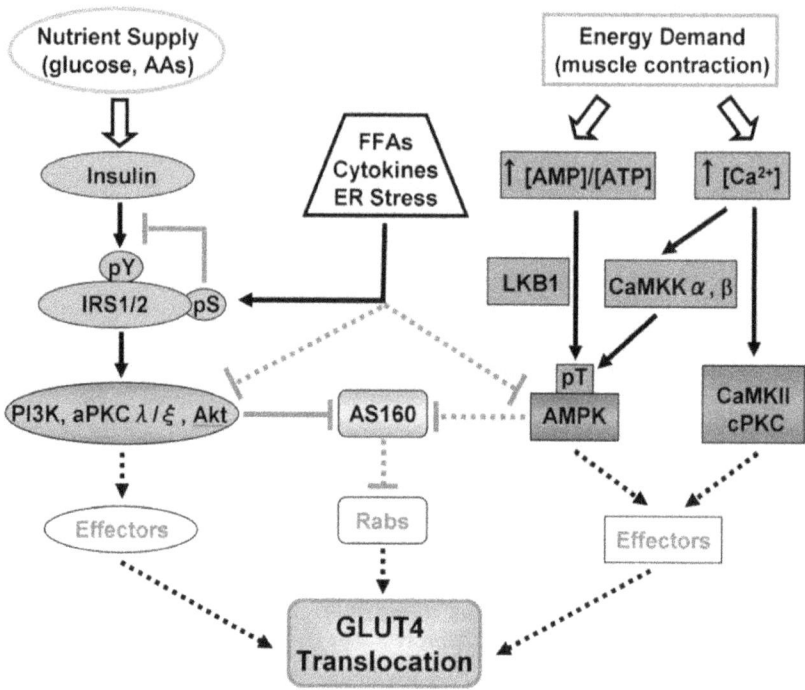

Figure 3. Convergence of signalling pathways: initiated by insulin and exercise leading to GLUT4 translocation insulin signalling through the PI 3-kinase pathway and muscle contraction through both elevated AMP/ATP ratios and intracellular [Ca^{2+}] leads to activation of downstream protein kinases (Akt, aPKCl/z, AMPK, CaMKII cPKC) that phosphorylate putative effectors that modulate steps in the GLUT4 trafficking pathways. Negative regulation of these pathways by fatty acids, cytokines, and endoplasmic reticulum stress responses are observed in obesity and diabetes, contributing to insulin resistance. Dashed lines imply hypothetical pathways not yet experimentally verified.

inhibitors of cellular metabolism, decreasing cellular energy supply and increasing AMP/ATP ratios (**Figure 3**) tend to increase glucose uptake by muscle cells. These effectors of glucose uptake are readily found in malaria infection as both a result of parasite and host mechanism for survival. In adipocytes and muscle cells, hyperosmotic stress, a common feature of SM, promote GLUT4 translocation by activating AMPK and Gab-1 dependent signalling pathway, respectively [44]. Furthermore, osmatic shock activates Akt substrates, which promotes GLUT4 exocytosis to the plasma membranes of adipocytes increasing glucose uptake [45] and in malaria, inducing hypoglycaemia. In a paradox of some sorts, chronic hyperosmotic stress causes insulin resistance in isolated or cultured adipocytes as shown by increased insulin concentration and hyperglycaemia. Apparently, mTOR signalling pathway arbitrates this hyperosmolality-induced hyperinsulinemia a phenomenon that has been observed in end stage SM disease in animals where a cycle of hyperglycaemia breeding more hyperosmolality leads to more insulin resistance [44]. An intricate mTOR signalling, involving an intricate negative feedback mechanism, aiming at insulin and AMPK signalling pathways have been revealed [46]. Further to that, GLUT4 compromised sensitivity to insulin signalling pathway is a common feature of obesity and diabetes mellitus mediated by fatty acids activity [47], cytokines activity [48] and endoplasmic reticulum stress response [49] (**Figure 3**). Activation of stress protein kinases that are involved in the phosphorylation of IRS proteins serine residues attenuate tyrosine phosphorylation of IRS by insulin causing the negative regulation of GLUT4 translocation to the plasma membrane surface (**Figure 3**). These processes are inimical to glucose homeostasis as does end stage non-reversible SM [15].

3. Glucose transporter I (GLUT1) and it involvement in malaria

Most cell depends on glucose as a key substrate for a variate of metabolic processes that are necessary for energy production and cellular building blocks. Transportation of glucose, and other carbohydrates, into the cytoplasm of most cells is through a 14 member family of integral membrane glucose transporter molecules also known as solute carrier 2A protein which are sub-divided into Classes I–III [50]. Within this superfamily is the glucose transporter 1 a Class I facilitative glucose transporter expressed in the hepatocytes [51] with the highest expression being found in the membrane of the erythrocyte or red blood cells (RBC's) [52] and also influences the glucose uptake across the blood brain barrier [53]. GLUT1 has various functions in the body amongst which being a receptor for the human T cell leukaemia virus [54] and glucose transport in T-cells where it regulates infection by the Human Immunodeficiency virus [55] appear to be the most prominent ones besides its involvement with malaria infection in both the red blood cell and the hepatocyte [55].

The malarial parasite expurgates a uni-directional trajectory during its infection of the human being from the time the *Plasmodium sporozoites* are injected into the bite by an infected mosquito to the period of overt symptomatic infection. After crossing the hepatic endothelium, sinusoids and entering the liver, sporozoites transverse several parenchymal liver cells before finally invading one in which the productive asymptomatic exoerythrocytic forms (EEF's) differentiation takes place with the origination thousands of RBC's-infective merozoites which are released into the circulation to start symptomatic infection [56].

Production of adenosine triphosphate (ATP) [24], the energy source of the blood stage merozoites and other erythrocytic stage parasites, is derived from glycolysis of which a model now exist for the *Plasmodium falciparum* [57] showing it as an equilibrated than an active process in the parasite [24]. GLUT1 has been shown to transport glucose from human plasma to the erythrocyte cytoplasm [58] from where the parasite encoded facilitative hexose transporter (PfHT) [59], which limits glucose entry into parasite's glycolysis [60]. Thus, the PfHT targeting in novel malaria treatment is plausible undertakings [61] seeing that in the murine malaria model, *P. berghei*, orthologous hexose transporter (PbHT), is expressed throughout the parasite's development in the mosquito vector, during hepatic and transmission stages [62]. When the PbHT are inhibited (by compound 3361), a drastic inhibition of growth of the hepatic parasitic stage of the *P. berghei* was observed, showing that glucose uptake is crucial in infected hepatocytes for both energy and nutrients supply for the parasite [61]. In vitro studies have established that the key parameters in the development of liver stage parasites were the glucose concentration in the cell culture media and utilisation of glucose by the Plasmodium liver stages [63]. Glucose requirements during the course of parasite development in the hepatocyte and the host cell molecular receptors involved with the uptake of glucose by the cells was studied in this work. *P. berghei* infection resulted in the depletion of ATP with subsequent translocation of GLUT1 from the cytoplasm to the membrane surface of infected hepatocytes which resulted in significantly higher glucose uptake compared to non-infected cells. Furthermore, glucose plays in a critical role during the development of the liver stage infection, modulating the Plasmodium development in the EEF's [52].

3.1. Effect of glucose on hepatic murine malaria infection model

Experiments have been carried out to the effect of glucose in the propagation of malaria disease in vitro and in vivo. Inclusion of various glucose from 1.25 to 20 mM in a hepatic cell (Huh7 cells) line which cover the physiological glucose concentration range, 2.5 to 10 mM [64], unravelled that the increasing glucose concentrations availability 48 hours post infection (hpi) correlated with overall *Plasmodium* patent infection [52]. Using a parasite load marker and cell viability, luminescence intensity [65], investigators reported that concentrations of glucose <10 mM, which is the cell medium standard, significantly impairs hepatic *Plasmodium* infection while excess glucose does not affect cell viability but is decreased at 2.5 and 1.5 mM glucose concentrations [52]. A flow cytometry-based approach using green fluorescent protein (GFP)-expressing *P. berghei* parasites [66] was used to determine the number of infected hepatic cells and parasite growth. The ability of parasite to transverse or invade hepatic cells was not dependent on glucose concentration within the initial 2 hours when sporozoites hepatocytes invasion was virtually complete [66], but after 48 hpi glucose concentration was important with concentrations of >20 mM showing the higher parasite development and lower at concentrations of glucose lower than glucose physiological range.

Furthermore, the parasite size correlates well with glucose concentration (very small parasites <50 μm^2 and fewer infected cells) while increasing glucose concentration (10–20 mM) favoured increased parasite sizes (>200 μm^2) and number of infected cells [52]. While hepatoma cells (Huh7 cells) depend highly on glucose uptake for ATP glycolysis synthesis [67], primary liver cells store glucose as glycogen from which ATP is obtained through oxidative phosphorylation. However, regardless of the hepatocyte source, parasite proliferation depends greatly on glucose concentration with increased glucose uptake highest in plasmodium-infected hepatocytes, parasite development and survival [52].

To demonstrate the link between hepatic stage parasite development, plasmodium replication and increased glucose uptake, fluorescent glucose analogue, 2-deoxy-2-[(7-nitro-2,1,3-benzoxadiazol-4-yl)amino]-D-glucose (2-NBDG) [68, 69], has been used. At 30 hpi set point and onward, significant glucose uptake by the hepatocyte and the parasite increases in cells infected by viable parasites as compared to non-infected cells and infected cells with non-replicating cells [52, 66].

Glucose uptake depends on several influences that include feeding and fasting status, exposure to heat or cold [70], physical activity [71], oxidative stress [72], hepatic diseases (steatosis, non-alcoholic fatty acid liver disease, hepatitis C virus infection) [73]. However, none of the stress-inducing factors contribute to the increase in glucose uptake besides the presence of malaria parasites in infected hepatocytes in any comparable measure which indicate Plasmodium parasite has a specific and unique way for handling glucose homeostasis.

Actually, experiments carried out have invariably shown that the malaria parasites induce glucose uptake that is not a non-specific response to stress or to infection but a specific and enhanced marked glucose uptake with a calculated end. Other intracellular organisms have been reported to have a dissimilar effect on glucose uptake which makes the *Plasmodium* glucose metabolism rather inimitable. *Toxoplasma gondii* does not depend on glucose uptake from the host [74]. On the other hand, cellular glucose uptake is suppressed through downregulation of cell surface glucose transporters expression during active hepatitis C virus replication [75]. This, then, characterises Plasmodium infection as an exceptional intracellular parasite glucose homeostasis machinery whose aetiology and mechanism of action has insidious connotations to human survival seeing that the parasites life cycle is intimately associated to and manipulates human biology at will.

3.2. Specific indications of GLUT1 implication in malarial parasite-infected-cell glucose uptake

In experiments that sought to ascertain by which specific glucose transporter was uptake enhancement possible, genes for the expression of 5 transmembrane glucose transporters were sequentially down-regulated and the effect of this measured in Huh& cell lines. Class I GLUT genes (GLUT1-4) and GLUT9, which is a HepG2 hepatoma cells (and Huh7 equivalent) glucose influx regulator [76], were screened for their influence of glucose uptake in malaria parasite-infected cells through silencing each gene at a time and determining the parasite load [52]. The GLUT1 gene knock down (KD) resulted in the most significant decrease in malaria parasites in these experiments. This did not only show that glucose uptake was important for parasite development but also that GLUT1 was responsible for the glucose uptake that causes enhanced parasite growth in the liver cells. Down-regulation of GKUT2, which the major glucose transporter in hepatocyte did not affect the glucose uptake in cells holding actively replicating parasites as it was observed that GLUT1 KD did not affect glucose uptake in non-infected cells [52]. Chemical inhibition of GLUT1 (adding 100 µM WZB117 to cell culture) in both hepatoma cells and primary hepatocytes has been reported as having the same decreased effect on glucose uptake, parasite development and replication as does GLUT1 KD.

3.3. Glucose transporter 1 expression in *Plasmodium*-infected cells

A hypothesis that the enhanced glucose uptake in *Plasmodium*-infected cells may due to an over expression of the GLUT1 in malaria is an intruding and tempting approach to explaining the increased glucose uptake that is associated with malarial hypoglycaemia. However, Meireles et al. [52] monitored the expression of the GLUT1 in infected Huh7 cells, at increasing time periods hpi, revealed a different and amazing phenomenon contrary to the hypothesis. No significant increase in GLUT1 mRNA was observed between infected and non-infected cells using fluorescence-activated cell sorting (FACS) technique [77] and analysing with quantitative real-time polymerase chain reaction (qPCR) and GLUT1 specific primers. This, therefore, means that the amplified glucose uptake by Plasmodium parasite-infected cells does not emanate from genetically induced GLUT1 synthesis but from the circulating pool of already existing glucose transporters.

As *Plasmodium* parasites increase in number in the infected cell, there is a proportional depletion of cytoplasmic ATP overall. It is necessary that GLUT1 to remain inactive during normal or reduced cellular energy demands or else it will derive hypoglycaemia. This necessary regulation occurs through the binding of ATP by GLUT1 cytoplasmic pockets [78] which causes conformational changes to the molecule inhibiting glucose transportation [79]. In a competitive binding principle, Adenosine monophosphate (AMP) and Adenosine diphosphate (ADP) counteract the ATP-induced conformational modulation by binding to the same site activating the glucose GLUT1-mediated transportation [78]. True enough, intracellular ATP has been reported to be significantly decreased in *Plasmodium* parasite-infected cells as compared to non-infected cells validating presumably decreased ATP/ADP/AMP ratio of malaria infection that drives conformational changes in GLUT1 [78–80]. The sequence of events in GLUT1 metabolism in malaria infection tends to follow a transcendence guided by the depletion of intracellular ATP, which activates the GLUT1 proteins and subsequent translocation to the infected cell membrane where it enhances glucose uptake driving the hypoglycaemia pathophysiology of malaria.

4. Comparison of GLUT1 and GLUT2 involvement in glucose uptake in malaria

The significant increase in infected liver cells through an enhanced action and translocation of GLUT1 to the surface membrane looks like the key mechanism by which Plasmodium parasites acquire the source of energy that is obligatory for their replication and survival. The ability to transport glucose across plasma membranes is a feature in most cells that make the hexose a ubiquitous common currency of metabolism [50]. Whereas GLUT2 represents the major glucose transporter, (uptake and release, in hepatocytes during the fed and starved state, respectively [50, 81], GLUT1 is also transcribed and expressed in the liver cells of the periportal and perivenular hepatic areas [82].

There are disparities between GLUT1 and GLUT2 in terms of their capacity to handle and affinity for glucose. GLUT2's capacity and affinity for glucose are inversely related, i.e. high capacity and low affinity shown by a Km value (glucose concentration at which transport is half of its maximum value) of 17 mM [83]. The Km value of GLUT1 is higher and much closer to that of the PfHT at 3 mM [83] as compared to 1 mM [23]. Therefore, GLUT1 may be better matched for hexose supply to the *Plasmodium* parasite in malarial hypoglycaemia where glucose concentration decreases towards the Km of the solute transporter.

There is a restriction of GLUT1 to membrane of liver cells that are proximal to the hepatic venule during basal states, although the transporter is expressed by all hepatocytes [50, 51, 82]. There is a decreasing gradient of oxygen and glucose as blood flows from the portal to hepatic venule due to the unidirectional perfusion of the hepatocyte plate [84]. This environment of reduced circulating glucose concentration [85] and hypoxia [86] are instrumental and conducive to the enhanced membranous expression of GLUT1. Hypoxia boosts liver stage malarial infection as much as does an activator of hypoxia inducible factor-1α (HIF-1α) or the hypoxia mimetic $CoCl_2$ [87]. On the other hand, increased concentrations of HIF-1α have been shown to upregulate GLUT1 expression [88] and $CoCl_2$ is known to enhance the translocation of the hexose transporter to the plasma membrane [52, 89]. Overall, GLUT1-mediated glucose transport seems to provide the important linkages defining the preferred tendency of *Plasmodium* parasites in infecting hypoxic hepatocytes and red blood cells or inducing hypoxia as a driver of enhanced infectivity.

5. Mode of action of GLUT1 in glucose transport

Consequent to the extensive replication of the Plasmodium parasite in hepatocyte is the depletion of intracellular glucose concentration and subsequently concentration of ATP as well. The compensatory mechanism is an increase in glucose uptake. This may either result from activation of GLUT1 transporters at cell membrane as a result of AMP-dependent conformational alterations or from the GLUT1 translocation to the plasma membranes towards parasite final development stages [52]. The resultant momentous increase in glucose uptake during malarial infection does not only affect *Plasmodium* infected cells. Non-infected cells within the immediate environ of the infected cells also experience a glucose and energy deficit that tends to trigger similar glucose uptakes, albeit at inferior response. A comparable slight decrease in intracellular ATP and increase in translocation of GLUT1 with concomitant slight increase in glucose uptake in non-infected cells although it is still not clear what mechanisms are involved in the regulation of GLUT1's translocation or activation [52]. Activation of pre-existing GLUT1 on the plasma membranes which enhance glucose uptake has been shown to be associated with stimulation of AMP-activated kinase activity [90]. Also, GLUT1 translocation to the plasma membrane has been shown to be prompted by insulin and ischaemia (GLUT4 too) [91] in a manner dependent on a phosphoinositide 3-kinase (PI3K) [92]. Captivatingly, down-regulation of the $\alpha1$ and $\alpha2$ subunits does not seem to affect parasite development and glucose uptake by parasite-infected cells [52]. Furthermore, insulin addition or inhibition of PI3K with Wortmannin [93] did not seem to have a negative effect on infection and infected cell glucose uptake [52]. Protein kinase C phosphorylation of GLUT1 generated rapid glucose uptake and heightened plasma membrane localization of GLUT1 [94]. Speculation that the same mechanism may be at play in malarial glucose transported is well supported as the inhibition of GLUT1 result in reduced parasite replication parasite general infectivity.

The liver should be considered as a major site for postprandial glucose removal seeing that it holds a volume to remove 30–40% of glucose existing after ingestion [95] which could mean a huge glucose supply necessitating uptake that will support parasite growth. The association between increased risk from malaria infection with P. falciparum and diabetes type 2 (DM 2) is emerging [96] which may link GLUT1 glucose uptake as a possible instigator in these disease common trajectory. Sub Saharan Africa has seen an upsurge in DM 2 [97] in an area where malaria has been endemic for several years. Plasmodium parasites from infected DM 2 individuals have also been shown to have a higher infective capacity than those from non-DM 2 individuals [98] showing possibly the uptake of glucose by parasite infected cells plays a critical role in rendering the parasites more potent in transmission of the disease. As such, GLUT1 may be a druggable target for the treatment of malaria. The modulation of GLUT1 in cells that contain the malaria parasite provides leads towards the use of energy supply inhibition as a potential weaponry in the arsenal to combat malaria.

6. Interactions of glycosylphosphatidylinositol glucose homeostasis in malaria

The molecular interactions that brings about the activation of GLUT1 either on the plasma membrane or in the cytoplasm has been directly linked to the decrease of glucose and subsequently ATP from within the cell. Depletion of either glucose or ATP is associated with an increase in parasite replication and maturation. However, the triggering of the events in the decrease in glucose and ATP should a *Plasmodium* parasite initiative as other intracellular parasites discussed do not have such an inherent mechanism of glucose homeostasis.

Glycosylphosphatidylinositol (GPI) belongs to a class of glycolipids that are ubiquitous in eukaryotes where they display a number of biological effects [99]. In parasites, GPI's are particularly abundant as free lipids or as anchors of proteins. The GPI also formulate the majority of glycoconjugates in the intraerythrocytic *P. falciparum* where it anchors to the cell membrane functionally important parasite proteins like the merozoite surface proteins (MSP-1, MSP-2, MSP-4) [100]. *P. falciparum* GPI synthesis is a developmental stage-specific manner which is crucial for development and survival of the parasite [101] in the same way GLUT1 recruitment has been discussed elsewhere. The parasite GPI mediates hypoglycaemia through an insulin mimetic activity in a manner that increases GLUT1 population of the molecule on the surface membrane of *Plasmodium* infected cells via a tyrosine kinase dependent signal transduction [102] which puts this molecule at the centre of the processes leading to glucose and ATP depletion in the infected cell.

The GPI has also been reported to drive the pathophysiology of malaria through the ability to induce proinflammatory cytokines in the host which include tumour necrosis factor (TNF-α), interleukin-1β (IL-1β), nitric oxide (NO), interferon-γ (IFN-γ) [19, 103]. There is an up-regulation of intercellular adhesion molecule-1, vascular cell adhesion molecule-1, and e-selectin expression in vascular endothelial cells and increases leukocyte and parasite cytoadherence via tyrosine kinase dependent signal transduction that has been observed [104]. Most of these synthetic processes where GPI is involved are energy dependent and expend ATP whose source is glucose thereby indivertibly upregulate demand for the hexose by most cells interactive with the anchoring molecule. There are structural similarities between insulin second messengers (phosphatidylinositol-PI) and *Plasmodium* GPI which makes the insulin memetic effect of the membrane anchored glycolipid induce hypoglycaemia [105, 106]. The structural similarity will entail the activation of steps for glucose uptake by-passing the insulin receptor (IR) position of insulin signal transduction system. With the numerous GPI production capacity of the Plasmodium parasite, there arises a multitude of cellular GLUT1 activation that give increased glucose uptake into the cells. This brings about increased glucose availability to the growing parasites.

To bring this into perspective the relationship between the GLUT1 transporters and the subsequent uptake of glucose uptake by the parasite, the glucose transporter in the parasite's role in final glucose utilisation by the parasite needs be explored.

7. Glucose transport in the intraerythrocytic *Plasmodium* parasites

With blood being a steady and abundant source of glucose, Plasmodium parasites find a haven and shelter of protection in the intraerythrocyte where they multiple and grow utilising glucose as the main energy source. When malarial parasites are deprived of glucose, ATP concentrations drop drastically and their hydrogen ion activity increased (pH drop) [107]. Parasite plasma membrane tend to depolarize with reduction in glucose concentration or reduced glycolysis or reduction of anaerobic fermentation of pyruvate to lactate, which are the systems by which parasites main sources of ATP [108]. Glycolysis provide faster ATP, although less efficient, than does oxidative phosphorylation at rates hundred times faster than the latter [109]. The malarial parasite does possess a glycolysis functionally disconnected branched TCA cycle which does not contribute to the Plasmodium energy homeostasis [110].

GLUT1, as mentioned elsewhere, delivers glucose to the cytoplasm of the RBC from the plasma in a passive down-a-concentration gradient facilitative process [111]. From the cell cytoplasm, the glucose has to transcend parasitophorous food vacuole (PFV) membrane which is highly porous to the solutes with molecular weights <1400 Da through high-capacity, low selectivity channels [112]. Uptake of glucose from the PFV is through a facilitative transport system carried out by, for *P. falciparum*, *Plasmodium falciparum* hexose transporter (PfHT) [PlasmaoDb accession number:PFB0210c] [24, 113].

There PfHT gene is a putative gene to the human glucose transporter gene with a homology to GLUT1. The predicted topology of PfHT protein has 12 transmembrane helices with both of its carboxy and amino terminals positioned in the cytoplasm of the cell (**Figure 4**). Functional characterisation of PfHT has shown that the parasite sugar transporter is a sodium-independent, saturable, facilitative hexose transporter [113] with a mechanistic difference with GLUT1 in the way it interacts with substrates [109]. Whereas PfHT transports D-glucose (Km-1 mM) and D-fructose (Km-11.5 mM), GLUT1 is selective for D-glucose (Km-2.4 mM). The affinity for glucose by PfHT, therefore means that the parasite may be acquire the hexose at very low plasma concentrations. This is also corroborated by the low Km of GLUT1, which transporter increases activity in infected cells, providing an efficient linkage between the infected and the parasite for glucose uptake. As shown in **Figure 4**, the unidirectional glucose uptake is favourable for parasite survival and maturation and can drive severe hypoglycaemia of severe malaria.

There has been a critical observation of hyperglycaemia occurring during severe malaria which has a penchant for fatal outcomes. In unpublished data, it has been observed that animals that develop hyperglycaemia with or without treatment or intervention tended to have adverse outcomes and hyperglycaemia in malaria was determined to be an end-point marker which required intervention. The molecular basis of hyperglycaemia development in a disease that hypoglycaemia is more of the norm than the exception finds its basis on a number of factors that include parasite infection, inflammatory host response and hormonal aberrations. These factors revolve around the gluconeogenesis and glycogenesis-glycogenolysis-glycolysis axis and how these play-out in malaria pathophysiology.

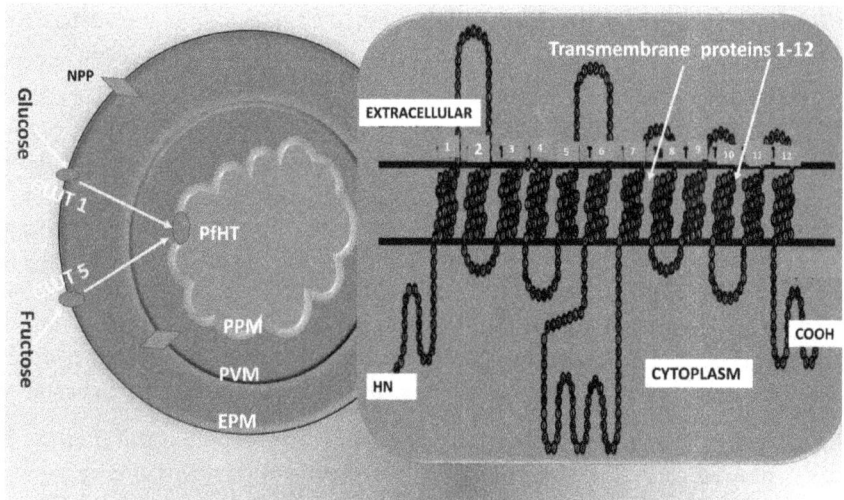

Figure 4. Hexoses uptake in Plasmodium-infected red blood cell shown in a schematic representation **A**. The EPM (erythrocyte plasma membrane), the PVM (parasitophorous vacuole membrane), the PPM (parasite plasma membrane) are shown. GLUT1, mammalian glucose transporter; GLUT5, mammalian fructose transporter; NPP, new permeability pathways (do not contribute significantly to the uptake of glucose [114]). **B** is the predicted topology of *Plasmodium falciparum* hexose transporter (PfHT) [113].

8. Production of glucose in malaria

Malaria has been associated with reduced glucose emanating from increased glucose utilisation by the growing intracellular parasites, especially towards the schizogony. Just as it has been shown that increased glucose trafficking is not as a result increased synthesis of GLUT1 but increased activation of the hexose transporter brought about depletion of ATP, there is no considerable doubt that there is increased glucose production in *P. falciparum* malaria which could be driven by the plasma hypoglycaemia. This same phenomenon was shown in adults infected with malaria that displayed increased glucose production [115].

Stimulation of gluconeogenesis is attributed to be the underlying reason for the increase in glucose production is severe malaria which leads to increased plasma glucose concentration. Concomitant with the rise in plasma glucose concentration is the rise in concentration of a hormone milieu comprising of plasma cortisol, glucagon and adiponectin. Surprisingly, the rise in the glucogenic hormones is not the cause of the increase in plasma glucose concentration.

In malaria, there is an increase in cytokine activities with TNF-α and IL-6 [116] which are known to have a stimulatory effect on glucose production indirectly through their influence on the secretion of glucose counter regulatory hormones [117]. Moreover, TNF-α stimulates the synthesis of prostaglandin synthesis by Kupffer cells and in turn, to complicate the picture somewhat, glucose production is inhibited by prostaglandin [117] showing an intricate mechanism involving glucose utilisation and production in severe malaria.

8.1. Malaria-related glucose clearance

Plasma glucose concentration is a balance between production and uptake or clearance which assist in the maintenance of the hexose within physiologic range. In cerebral malaria, showing severe malaria, there is an increase of glucose clearance rate by 42% and to a lesser extent in uncomplicated malaria increased by 9%. However, the overwhelming determinant of plasma glucose concentration in malaria is not through increased or decreased production but it is presumed to be through increased peripheral glucose uptake [115]. In theory, infected red blood cells have an increased glucose consumption of between 30 and 75 times than non-infected erythrocytes up to the time of trophozoite development of the parasite [118]. Increased glucose and lactate kinetics [6] and alanine metabolism have been reported in acute falciparum malaria [119]. The environmental stressor phenomenon brought about malarial illness impinges negatively on glucose utilisation with the overt outcome of glucose impaired metabolic processes like glycogenolysis and gluconeogenesis.

8.2. Malarial glycogenolysis

The glycogen mass in muscle and liver of infected animals has been observed to be much less as compared to control animals exposed to the same amount of food and water. Generally, the rate of glycogenesis in malaria is slow to absent as it is overridden by the quest to maintain euglycaemia in the face of hypoglycaemic threats and pressures. Glycogenolysis or glycogen breakdown to yield plasma glucose has more capacity than glycogenesis in both the liver and the muscles, however this occurrence may not cause hypoglycaemic tendencies of malaria. There is a hepatic autoregulation in as far as glycogen content is concerned in malaria, but its contribution to malarial hypoglycaemia is limited as compared to the increased clearance of glucose in malaria. Furthermore, glycogen, although lower in content in infected cases as compared to non-infected cases, is always present and not depleted completely in malaria [120].

8.3. Malarial gluconeogenesis

There has been a remarkable observation that, gluconeogenesis tends to increase with severity of the disease in *P. falciparum* infection and the more severe the disease the higher the stimulation degree. The previous consensus has been to the contrary of this observation in both pregnant and non-pregnant women with impaired gluconeogenesis as a recognised paradigm in malaria [121, 122]. The increased gluconeogenic stimulation is premised on the very important gluconeogenic precursor, the amino acid glutamine [123]. Children with acute malaria tend to have low concentrations of the amino acid [124] and will result in an increase rate of gluconeogenesis in a negative feedback mechanism rather than cause impairment. Furthermore, glycerol metabolism remains intact in malaria [125] and making the increase in gluconeogenic activity an perpetual enigma as fatty acid metabolism is also of no consequent in the aetiology of the glucose production process. Supply of gluconeogenic precursors, soluble chemical mediators and counterregulatory hormones remain key protagonists in the increases gluconeogenesis of malaria although none of these is directly involved in the process. The paracrine hormones overture seems also a critical but complicated avenue in explaining the increased gluconeogenic activity seen in malaria as there have a close influence on classical counterregulatory hormones and as well as on themselves. When prostaglandins synthesis, for instance, is inhibited, there is a subsequent rise in glucose production in healthy individuals [126].

In the liver, Kupffer cells the major producer of prostaglandins [117], have high concentrations of the malaria pigment which elicit prostaglandin synthesis, tend towards hyperplastic production of the inflammatory mediators synthesis [127] in subjects with severe malaria [128]. This impairment of Kupffer cell function brings about the concomitant intrahepatic autoregulation loss of the glucose homeostasis. The severity of Kupffer cells dysfunctionality will determine the degree of disturbances in gluconeogenesis. Maximum stimulation of gluconeogenesis is invariably inhibited by intrahepatic factors in uncomplicated malaria cases. As a result, changes in the rate of gluconeogenesis become paramount in chronic adaptation to glucose demand while glycogenosis rates carter for adaptations to acute changes in glucose utilisation of developmental trophozoite stages.

Gluconeogenesis is much more stimulated in cerebral malaria as compared to non-complicated malaria. Therefore, the Kupffer cell-liver parenchymal cell interaction functions at a dual level comprising of an acute stage for emergency situations which regulates the glycogen content while the chronic level monitors gluconeogenesis. The glucose homeostasis regulating hormones respond to the either the acute effects, i.e. insulin, glucagon catecholamines, or the chronically following a delay, i.e. cortisol and growth hormone. With these hormonal controls, the duality of acute-chronic effects within the Kupffer cell-hepatocyte interactions are under the influence of wider and complex products that are produced by both cell types. In essence the hormonal interactions in the Kupffer cell influences the closely related functions in the hepatocyte and vice versa.

The synthesis of glucose by the liver involves the delivery of substrates and a gluconeogenesis pathway that is intact and functional. Gluconeogenesis may be selectively impaired by alanine supply to the liver. In severe malaria, decreased blood flow to the liver [129] as well as hepatocyte dysfunction [130] may play a role in the impairment of alanine delivery to the liver consequently affecting gluconeogenesis [119]. There is a difference in the ability of reduced alanine supply to the liver in influencing gluconeogenesis that is not experienced with glycerol or glutamine [21]. This is mainly due to two of many possible causes, one which is physiological and another analytical. Glutamine and glycerol are converted to glucose may occur in the liver and the kidney as well while glucose synthesis from alanine is mainly confined to the liver. Furthermore, the measurement of glucose metabolism using stable isotopes does not discriminate hepatic and kidney gluconeogenesis [123]. Regardless, the complexity of these interactions is further intricated by the endocrinological function of the adipose tissue and its influence on both liver and muscle cell types but the increase in gluconeogenesis in malaria remains a fundamental fact.

9. Free fatty acids (FFAs) in malarial glucose regulation

While data in literature about FFAs in malaria seem conflicting, elevated plasma concentration of FFAs and triacylglycerols have been reported in acute malaria amongst adult subjects [131, 132] and in children too [128]. However, evidence exists on the absence of change in plasma concentrations of FFAs over prolonged fast in malaria patients [133]. Actually, in vitro data has shown a stimulation of lipogenesis and inhibition of lipolysis by malaria products [134]. In normal human beings an increase in glucose concentration has a tendency to suppress adipocytes lipolysis [135]. However, it is still not clear whether an increase of glucose in malaria will have the same effect. There has been a constant finding that high-density and low-density lipoproteins were lower in malaria cases as compared to controls and triacylg-lycerols were higher as compared to normal controls but without statistical significance when compared to controls displaying some symptoms e.g. fibrillations [135]. In acute malaria, plasma glucose has been shown to remain significantly elevated even when plasma FFAs are no longer increased [132]. Hepatic autoregulation is defined by an acute increase in FFAs which stimulates gluconeogenesis, to replenish depleted glycolysis intermediates, [136] and decrease glycogenesis [137, 138] with glucose production remaining the same [136, 138–140]. Hepatic autoregulation of glucose metabolism is attributed to both intrahepatic and extrahepatic. Ultimately, the autoregulatory mechanism rest on the decrease of liver glycogenolysis facilitated by insulin secretion to counteract FFAs stimulatory effects on glucose production during fasting. Hepatic glycogen content plays a regulatory role in glycogenolysis such that in malaria, where there is a low glycogen content, it is expected that there is no effect of FFAs on extrahepatic regulation [141].

10. Malaria treatment and glucose metabolism

Paroxysms of fever are usually the classical presentation of *P. falciparum* induced malaria. The febrile paroxysms are generally associated with shaking chills, profuse sweating, headache, rigours, fatigue, arthralgia, back ache, abdominal pain, nausea with vomiting, diarrhoea and at times prehepatic jaundice [142]. Atypical manifestations of malaria are more common as most classical symptoms are observed in a section of the malaria infected individuals (50–70%). In severe cases of malaria (SM) patients may present with cerebral malaria (CM), cerebellar ataxia or multiple seizures, hypoglycaemic seizures, cerebral malaria, acute kidney injury, severe malaria anaemia (SMA), thrombocytopaenia, haemoglobinuria, noncardiogenic pulmonary oedema, acute respiratory disease syndrome/ acute respiratory lung injury and other related conditions [143]. Hyperglycaemia is also a prominent finding, although usually missed, in malaria through increased glucose production and possibly insulin resistance driven by the proinflammatory mediatory common in malaria [144]. The hyperglycaemia may invariably lead to non-ketotic hyperosmolar hyperglycaemia state shock with higher fatal outcomes as compared to normoglycaemic individuals [26]. Therefore, treatment should be aimed at alleviating these manifestations more in malaria as well as the parasite. However, major treatment regimens are anti-parasitic than they are anti-disease. An association of hyperglycaemia, severe malaria and CM has been observed to have more fatal outcomes as there is a high glucose production stimulation [145]. However, the hyperglycaemic cases have been staccato in nature with reports of one or two cases out of many cases [146].

Various anti-malarial agents have been used for the treatment of malaria with some having negative effect on glucose homeostasis. These include the use hydroxychloroquine, hydroquinolones, artemisinin and its derivatives. Experimental malaria treatment has been reported with a range of phytochemicals coming into use which showed preservation of glucose homeostasis bearing in mind that some of the phototherapeutics have anti-inflammatory activities that may influences insulin resistance of malaria [147]. The effect of quinine and other quinolones on hypoglycaemia has been reported by many investigators and will not be covered here. The use of asiatic acid and other triterpenes is an area that is emerging in the fight against malaria. Glucose homeostasis during administration of the phytochemicals in malaria is given below:

10.1. Asiatic acid (AA) and glucose homeostasis in malaria

In streptozotocin (STZ)-induced diabetic rats, AA has been shown to have an anti-diabetic effect where it mediates glycogenolysis and release of glucose for glycolysis [148]. Hypoglycaemia development in malaria has been attributed to anti-malarial agents like quinine and hydroxychloroquine which displays hyperinsulinemia effects [149]. The triad of hypoglycaemia, hyperlactaemia and non-respiratory acidosis (nRA) are associated with elevated concomitantly in diseases that are not associated with malaria and AA has been shown to alleviate such conditions through inhibition of pro-inflammatory mediators like TNF-α [150]. The causal relationship that exists between deranged glucose homeostasis and malaria is linked through TNF-α [151]. Even in diseases such as *Borrelia recurrentis*, the triumvirate of hypoglycaemia, nRA and hyperlactaemia is present showing that the inflammatory response is involved [152]. AA has both an anti-parasitic and anti-disease effect in malaria [5, 8, 9, 13]. It has been shown that AA influences glucose metabolism and this could be through its effect on the inhibition of soluble inflammatory mediators such TNF-α [8]. Associated with this glucose homeostasis attenuation by AA was also an observable effect of the phytochemical on the hormonal milieu in malaria [8]. Together with an anti-parasitic activity, AA has anti-hyperglycaemic, antioxidant, pro-oxidant properties that are essential for glucose metabolism and has been shown to attenuate key glycolytic enzymes in diabetes mellitus as well as in murine malaria [8, 153].

On the hormonal modulation aspect, AA influences glucagon effects on food and water intake and weight in that it terminates the satiate and anorexic effect of the hormone when in high concentrations as in malaria [154]. AA oral administration has also been shown to ablate hyperlactaemia, which is a product of malaria induced-hypoxia, resulting in the wellbeing of the experimental animals not seen in the malaria infected non-treated animals [155].

The carbohydrate metabolic influence and anti-inflammatory effect of AA has been observed and this makes the phytopharmaceutical's ability to attenuate nRA, hyperlactatemia and hypoglycaemia in malaria possible [8]. The transient and fatal hyperglycaemia observed in end-stage malaria and driven by inflammation-induced insulin resistance may be ameliorated by the administration of AA through its anti-hyperglycaemic and immunologic effect.

11. Conclusion

Malaria syndrome vacillates between different events occurring concurrently or in episodes of dissimilar presentations of which glucose homeostatic dysfunction is a prominent one. Hypoglycaemia is driven by an increased consumption of energy which causes the activation of GLUT1 glucose transporters causing increased glucose uptake into both the infected and uninfected cell. PfHT supplies glucose to growing parasite exacerbating hypoglycaemia. Hyperglycaemia, hypoglycaemia, hyperlactaemia and hyperinsulinemia are facets of the syndrome in contention for supremacy in malaria which other forms of malarial treatment tend to promote. Asiatic acid and other similar phytochemical with known pleiotropic effects promise to provide anti-parasitic and anti-disease effect in malaria.

Conflict of interest

Authors declare no conflict of interest.

Author details

Greanious Alfred Mavondo[1]*, Joy Mavondo[2], Wisdom Peresuh[3], Mary Dlodlo[1] and Obadiah Moyo[4]

*Address all correspondence to: greaniousa@gmail.com and greanious.mavondo@nust.ac.zw

1 National University of Science and Technology (NUST), Faculty of Medicine, Pathology Department, Mpilo Hospital NUST, Bulawayo, Zimbabwe

2 Imagagate Diagnostics, c/o Dalony Distributors, Bulawayo, Zimbabwe

3 Labnet Laboratories, Bulawayo, Zimbabwe

4 Chitungwiza General Hospital, Harare, Zimbabwe

References

[1] D'Alessandro U, Ubben D, Hamed K, Ceesay SJ, Okebe J, Taal M, et al. Malaria in infants aged less than six months-Is it an area of unmet medical need? Malaria Journal. 2012;**11**:400. Available from: http://www.malariajournal.com/content/11/1/400

[2] Doolan DL, Dobaň C, Baird JK. Acquired immunity to malaria. Clinical Microbiology Reviews. 2009;**22**(1):13-36. DOI: 10.1128/CMR.00025-08

[3] WHO. Severe falciparum malaria. Communicable diseases cluster. Transactions of the Royal Society of Tropical Medicine and Hygiene. 2000;**94**:1-90

[4] Cox J, Hay SI, Abeku TA, Checchi F, Snow RW. The uncertain burden of *Plasmodium falciparum* epidemics in Africa. Trends in Parasitology. 2007;**23**:142-148

[5] Mavondo GA, Mkhwananzi BN, Mabandla MV, Musabayane CT. Asiatic acid influences parasitaemia reduction and ameliorates malaria anaemia in *P. berghei* infected Sprague-Dawley male rats. BMC Complementary and Alternative Medicine. 2016;**16**(1):357. DOI: 10.1186/s12906-016-1338-z

[6] Agbenyega T, Angus BJ, Bedu-Addo G, Baffoe-Bonnie B, Guyton T, Stacpoole PW, et al. Glucose and lactate kinetics in children with severe malaria. The Journal of Clinical Endocrinology and Metabolism. 2000;**85**:1569-1576

[7] Binh TQ, Davis TM, Johnston W, Thu LT, Boston R, Danh PT, et al. Glucose metabolism in severe malaria: Minimal model analysis of the intravenous glucose tolerance test incorporating a stable glucose label. Metabolism. 1997;**46**:1435-1440

[8] Mavondo GA, Mkhwananzi BN, Mabandla MV, Musabayane CT. Asiatic acid influences glucose homeostasis in *P. berghei* murine malaria infected Sprague Dawley rats. African Journal of Traditional, Complementary, and Alternative Medicines. 2016;**13**(5):91-101. DOI: 10.21010/ajtcam.v13i5.13

[9] Mavondo GA, Musabayane CT. Transdermal drug delivery of asiatic acid influences renal function and electrolyte handling in *Plasmodium berghei*-infected Sprague-Dawley male rats. Journal of Diseases and Medicinal Plants. 2018;**4**(1):18-29. DOI: 10.11648/j.jdmp.20180401.13

[10] Mavondo GA. Malaria disease perspective and an opinion: Should malaria treatment target the parasite or the malarial pathophysiology generated by the parasite or both? EC Microbiology. 2017;**7**(5):149-154

[11] Davis TM, Binh TQ, Thu le TA, Long TT, Johnston W, Robertson K, et al. Glucose and lactate turnover in adults with *falciparum* malaria: Effect of complications and antimalarial therapy. Transactions of the Royal Society of Tropical Medicine and Hygiene. 2002;**96**:411-417

[12] Mavondo GA, Kasvosve I. Antimalarial phytochemicals: Delineation of the triterpene asiatic acid malarial anti-disease and pathophysiological remedial activities-part II. Journal of Infectious Disease and Pathology. 2017;**1**:103

[13] Mavondo GA, Kasvosve I. Antimalarial phytochemicals: Delineation of the triterpene asiatic acid malarial anti-disease and pathophysiological remedial activities-part I. Journal of Infectious Disease and Pathology. 2017;**1**:104

[14] Mavondo GA, Musabayane CT. Asiatic acid-pectin hydrogel matrix patch transdermal delivery system influences parasitaemia suppression and inflammation reduction in *P. berghei* murine malaria infected Sprague-Dawley rats. Asian Pacific Journal of Tropical Medicine. 2016;**9**(12):1172-1180. DOI: 10.1016/j.apjtm.2016.10.008

[15] Eltahir EM, ElGhazali1 G, A-Elgadir TME, A-Elbasit IE, Elbashir MI, Giha1 HA. Raised plasma insulin level and homeostasis model assessment (HOMA) score in cerebral malaria: Evidence for insulin resistance and marker of virulence. Acta Biochimica Polonica. 2010;**57**(4):513-520

[16] English M, Sauerwein R, Waruiru C, Mosobo M, Obiero J, Lowe B, et al. Acidosis in severe childhood malaria. The Quarterly Journal of Medicine. 1997;**90**:263-270

[17] Maier AG, Rug M, O'Neill MT, Brown M, Chakravorty S, Szestak T, et al. Exported proteins required for virulence and rigidity of *Plasmodium falciparum*-infected human erythrocytes. Cell. 2008;**134**:48-61

[18] Maier AG, Cooke BM, Cowman AF, Tilley L. Malaria parasite proteins that remodel the host erythrocyte. Nature Reviews. 2009;7:341-354

[19] Moxon CA, Grau GE, Craig AG. Malaria: Modification of the red blood cell and consequences in the human host. British Journal of Haematology. 2011;154:670-679. DOI: 0.1111/j.1365-2141.2011.08755.x

[20] Cowman AF, Crabb BS. Invasion of red blood cells by malaria parasites. Cell. 2006;124:755-766. DOI: 10.1016/j.cell.2006.02.006

[21] Dekker E, Hellerstein M, Romijn JA, Neese RA, Peshu N, Endert E, et al. Glucose homeostasis in children with *Falciparum* malaria: Precursor supply limits gluconeogenesis and glucose production. Journal of Clinical Endocrinology and Metabolism. 1997;82(8): 2514-1521. DOI: 10.1210/jc.82.8.2514

[22] Krishna S, Woodrow CJ, Burchmore RJ, Saliba KJ, Kirk K. Hexose transport in asexual stages of *Plasmodium falciparum* and kinetoplastidae. Parasitology Today. 2000;16:516-521

[23] Woodrow CJ, Burchmore RJ, Krishna S. Hexose permeation pathways in *Plasmodium falciparum*-infected erythrocytes. Proceedings of the National Academy of Sciences of the United States of America. 2000;29:9931-9936

[24] Kirk K, Horner HA, Kirk J. Glucose uptake in *Plasmodium falciparum*-infected erythrocytes is an equilibrative not an active process. Molecular and Biochemical Parasitology. 1996;82:195-205

[25] Giha HA, Elghazali G, A-Elgadir TM, A-Elbasit IE, Eltahir EM, Baraka OZ, et al. Clinical pattern of severe *Plasmodium falciparum* malaria in Sudan in an area characterized by seasonal and unstable malaria transmissio. Transactions of the Royal Society of Tropical Medicine and Hygiene. 2005;99:243-251

[26] Osier FH, Berkley JA, Ross A, Sanderson F, Mohammed S, Newton CR. Abnormal blood glucose concentrations on admission to a rural Kenyan district hospital: Prevalence and outcome. Archives of Disease in Childhood. 2003;88:621-625

[27] Wood IS, Trayhurn P. Glucose transporters (GLUT and SGLT): Expanded families of sugar transport proteins. The British Journal of Nutrition. 2003;89(7):3-9

[28] Hruz PW, Mueckler MM. Structural analysis of the GLUT1 facilitative glucose transporter (review). Molecular Membrane Biology. 2001;18:183-193

[29] Tsirigos KD, Peters C, Shu N, Käll L, Elofsson AT. The TOPCONS web server for consensus prediction of membrane protein topology and signal peptides. Nucleic Acids Research. 2015;43:W401-W407

[30] Stuart CA, Wen G, Gustafson WC, Thompson EA. Comparison of GLUT1, GLUT3, and GLUT4 mRNA and the subcellular distribution of their proteins in normal human muscle. Metabolism. 2000;49:1604-1609

[31] Stuart CA, Yin D, Howell ME, Dykes RJ, Laffan JJ, Ferrando AA. Hexose transporter mRNAs for GLUT4, GLUT5, and GLUT12 predominate in human muscle. American Journal of Physiology. Endocrinology and Metabolism. 2006;291:E1067-E1073

[32] Wood IS, Hunter L, Trayhurn P. Expression of Class III facilitative glucose transporter genes (GLUT-10 and GLUT-12) in mouse and human adipose tissues. Biochemical and Biophysical Research Communications. 2003;**308**:43-49

[33] Bryant NJ, Govers R, James DE. Regulated transport of the glucose transporter GLUT4. Nature Reviews. Molecular Cell Biology. 2002;**3**:267-277

[34] Al-Hasani H, Kunamneni RK, Dawson K, Hinck CS, Muller-Wieland D, Cushman SW. Roles of the N- and C-termini of GLUT4 in endocytosis. Journal of Cell Science. 2002; **115**:131-140

[35] Sandoval IV, Martinez-Arca S, Valdueza J, Palacios S, Holman GD. Distinct reading of different structural determinants modulates the dileucine-mediated transport steps of the lysosomal membrane protein LIMPII and the insulin-sensitive glucose transporter GLUT4. The Journal of Biological Chemistry. 2000;**275**:39874-39885

[36] Martinez-Arca S, Lalioti VS, Sandoval IV. Intracellular targeting and retention of the glucose transporter GLUT4 by the perinuclear storage compartment involves distinct carboxyl-tail motifs. Journal of Cell Science. 2000;**113**:1705-1715

[37] Huang S, Czech MP. The GLUT4 glucose transporter. Cell Metabolism Review. 2007;**5**:237-252

[38] Herman MA, Kahn BB. Glucose transport and sensing in the maintenance of glucose homeostasis and metabolic harmony. The Journal of Clinical Investigation. 2006;**116**: 1767-1775

[39] Rose AJ, Richter EA. Skeletal muscle glucose uptake during exercise: How is it regulated? Physiology (Bethesda). 2005;**20**:260-270

[40] Thong FS, Dugani CB, Klip A. Turning signals on and off: GLUT4 traffic in the insulin-signaling highway. Physiology (Bethesda). 2005;**20**:271-284

[41] Watson RT, Kanzaki M, Pessin JE. Regulated membrane trafficking of the insulin-responsive glucose transporter 4 in adipocytes. Endocrine Reviews. 2004;**25**:177-204

[42] Jiang ZY, Chawla A, Bose A, Way M, Czech MP. A phosphatidylinositol 3-kinase-independent insulin signaling pathway to N-WASP/Arp2/3/F-actin required for GLUT4 glucose transporter recycling. The Journal of Biological Chemistry. 2003;**277**:509-515

[43] Tang X, Powelka AM, Soriano NA, Czech MP, Guilherme A. PTEN, but not SHIP2, suppresses insulin signaling through the phosphatidylinositol 3-kinase/Akt pathway in 3T3–L1 adipocytes. The Journal of Biological Chemistry. 2005;**280**:22523-22529

[44] Gual P, Gonzalez T, Gremeaux T, Barres R, Le Marchand-Brustel Y, Tanti JF. Hyperosmotic stress inhibits insulin receptor substrate-1 function by distinct mechanisms in 3T3–L1 adipocytes. The Journal of Biological Chemistry. 2003;**278**:26550-26557

[45] Sbrissa D, Shisheva A. Acquisition of unprecedented phosphatidylinositol 3, 5-bisphosphate rise in hyperosmotically stressed 3T3–L1 adipocytes, mediated by ArPIKfyve-PIKfyve pathway. The Journal of Biological Chemistry. 2005;**280**:7883-7889

[46] Um SH, D'Alessio D, Thomas G. Nutrient overload, insulin resistance, and ribosomal protein S6 kinase 1, S6K1. Cell Metabolism. 2006;**3**:393-402

[47] Kim JK, Fillmore JJ, Sunshine MJ, Albrecht B, Higashimori T, Kim DW, et al. PKC-theta knockout mice are protected from fat-induced insulin resistance. The Journal of Clinical Investigation. 2004;**114**:823-827

[48] Weisberg SP, McCann D, Desai M, Rosenbaum M, Leibel RL, Ferrante Jr AW. Obesity is associated with macrophage accumulation in adipose tissue. The Journal of Clinical Investigation. 2003;**112**:1796-1808

[49] Ozcan U, Yilmaz E, Ozcan L, Furuhashi M, Vaillancourt E, Smith RO, et al. Chemical chaperones reduce ER stress and restore glucose homeostasis in a mouse model of type 2 diabetes. Science. 2006;**313**:1137-1140

[50] Mueckler M, Thorens B. The SLC2 (GLUT) family of membrane transporters. Molecular Aspects of Medicine. 2013;**34**:121-138

[51] Tal M, Schneider DL, Thorens B, Lodish HF. Restricted expression of the erythroid/brain glucose transporter isoform to perivenous hepatocytes in rats modulation by glucose. The Journal of Clinical Investigation. 1990;**86**:986-992

[52] Meireles P, Sales-Dias J, Andrade CM, Mello-Vieira J, Mancio-Silva L, Simas JP, et al. GLUT1-mediated glucose uptake plays a crucial role during *Plasmodium* hepatic infection. Cellular Microbiology. 2017;**19**(2):e12646

[53] Koranyi L, Bourey RE, James D, Mueckler M, Fiedorek Jr FT, Permutt MA. Glucose transporter gene expression in rat brain: Pretranslational changes associated with chronic insulin-induced hypoglycemia, fasting, and diabetes. Molecular and Cellular Neurosciences. 1991;**2**:244-225

[54] Manel N, Kim FJ, Kinet S, Taylor N, Sitbon M, Battini JL. The ubiquitous glucose transporter GLUT-1 is a receptor for HTLV. Cell. 2003;**115**:449-459

[55] Loisel-Meyer S, Swainson L, Craveiro M, Oburoglu L, Mongellaz C, Costa C. Glut 1-mediated glucose transport regulates HIV infection. Proceedings of the National Academy of Sciences of the United States of America. 2012;**109**:2549-2554

[56] Prudencio M, Rodriguez A, Mota MM. The silent path to thousands of merozoites: The *Plasmodium* liver stage. Nature Reviews. Microbiology. 2006;**4**:849-856

[57] Penkler G, du Toit F, Adams W, Rautenbach M, Palm DC, van Niekerk DD, et al. Construction and validation of a detailed kinetic model of glycolysis in *Plasmodium falciparum*. The FEBS Journal. 2015;**282**:1481-1511

[58] Hellwig B, Joost HG. Differentiation of erythrocyte-(GLUT1), liver-(GLUT2), and adipocyte-type (GLUT4) glucose transporters by binding of the inhibitory ligands cytochalasin B, forskolin, dipyridamole, and isobutylmethylxanthine. Molecular Pharmacology. 1991;**40**:383-389

[59] Joet T, Eckstein-Ludwig U, Morin C, Krishna S. Validation of the hexose transporter of *Plasmodium falciparum* as a novel drug target. Proceedings of the National Academy of Sciences of the United States of America. 2003;**100**:7476-7479

[60] Tjhin ET, Staines HM, van Schalkwyk DA, Krishna S, Saliba KJ. Studies with the *Plasmodium falciparum* hexokinase reveal that PfHT limits the rate of glucose entry into glycolysis. FEBS Letters. 2013;**587**:3182-3187

[61] Slavic K, Delves MJ, Prudencio M, Talman AM, Straschil U, Derbyshire ET. Use of a selective inhibitor to define the chemotherapeutic potential of the plasmodial hexose transporter in different stages of the parasite's life cycle. Antimicrobial Agents and Chemotherapy. 2011;**55**:2824-2830

[62] Slavic K, Straschil U, Reininger L, Doerig C, Morin C, Tewari R, et al. Life cycle studies of the hexose transporter of *Plasmodium* species and genetic validation of their essentiality. Molecular Microbiology. 2010;**75**:1402-1413

[63] Itani S, Torii M, Ishino T. D-Glucose concentration is the key factor facilitating liver stage maturation of *Plasmodium*. Parasitology International. 2014;**63**:584-590

[64] Shrayyef MZ, Gerich JE. Normal glucose homeostasis. In: Poretsky L, editor. Principles of Diabetes Mellitus. Berlin, Germany: Springer; 2010

[65] Ploemen IH, Prudencio M, Douradinha BG, Ramesar J, Fonager J, van Gemert GJ. Visualisation and quantitative analysis of the rodent malaria liver stage by real time imaging. PLoS One. 2009;**4**:e7881

[66] Prudencio M, Rodrigues CD, Ataide R, Mota MM. Dissecting in vitro host cell infection by *Plasmodium* sporozoites using flow cytometry. Cellular Microbiology. 2008;**10**:218-224

[67] Kroemer G, Pouyssegur J. Tumor cellmetabolism: Cancer's Achilles' heel. Cancer Cell. 2008;**13**:472-482

[68] O'Neil RG, Wu L, Mullani N. Uptake of a fluorescent deoxyglucose analog (2-NBDG) in tumor cells. Molecular Imaging and Biology. 2005;**7**:388-392

[69] Yamada K, Saito M, Matsuoka H, Inagaki N. A real-time method of imaging glucose uptake in single, living mammalian cells. Nature Protocols. 2007;**2**:753-762

[70] Cunningham JJ, Gulino MA, Meara PA, Bode HH. Enhanced hepatic insulin sensitivity and peripheral glucose uptake in cold acclimating rats. Endocrinology. 1985;**117**:1585-1589

[71] Pencek RR, James FD, Lacy DB, Jabbour K, Williams PE, Fueger PT, et al. Exercise-induced changes in insulin and glucagon are not required for enhanced hepatic glucose uptake after exercise but influence the fate of glucose within the liver. Diabetes. 2004;**53**:3041-3047

[72] Bitar MS, Al-Saleh E, Al-Mulla F. Oxidative stress-mediated alterations in glucose dynamics in a genetic animal model of type II diabetes. Life Sciences. 2005;**77**:2552-2573

[73] Yu JW, Sun LJ, Liu W, Zhao YH, Kang P, Yan BZ. Hepatitis C virus core protein induces hepatic metabolism disorders through down-regulation of the SIRT1-AMPK signaling pathway. International Journal of Infectious Diseases. 2013;**17**:e539-e545

[74] Blume M, Rodriguez-Contreras D, Landfear S, Fleige T, Soldati-Favre D, Lucius R, et al. Hostderived glucose and its transporter in the obligate intracellular pathogen *Toxoplasma gondii* are dispensable by glutaminolysis. Proceedings of the National Academy of Sciences of the United States of America. 2009;**106**:12998-13003

[75] Kasai D, Adachi T, Deng L, Nagano-Fujii M, Sada K, Ikeda M. HCV replication suppresses cellular glucose uptake through down-regulation of cell surface expression of glucose transporters. Journal of Hepatology. 2009;**50**:883-894

[76] Takanaga H, Chaudhuri B, Frommer WB. GLUT1 and GLUT9 as major contributors to glucose influx in HepG2 cells identified by a high sensitivity intramolecular FRET glucose sensor. Biochimica et Biophysica Acta. 2008;**1778**:1091-1099

[77] Albuquerque SS, Carret C, Grosso AR, Tarun AS, Peng X, Kappe SH. Host cell transcriptional profiling during malaria liver stage infection reveals a coordinated and sequential set of biological events. BMC Genomics. 2009;**10**:270

[78] Blodgett DM, De Zutter JK, Levine KB, Karim P, Carruthers A. Structural basis of GLUT1 inhibition by cytoplasmic ATP. The Journal of General Physiology. 2007;**130**:157-168

[79] Levine KB, Cloherty EK, Fidyk NJ, Carruthers A. Structural and physiologic determinants of human erythrocyte sugar transport regulation by adenosine triphosphate. Biochemistry. 1998;**37**:12221-12232

[80] Cloherty EK, Diamond DL, Heard KS, Carruthers A. Regulation of GLUT1-mediated sugar transport by an antiport/uniport switch mechanism. Biochemistry. 1996;**35**:13231-13239

[81] Thorens B, Cheng ZQ, Brown D, Lodish HF. Liver glucose transporter: A basolateral protein in hepatocytes and intestine and kidney cells. The American Journal of Physiology. 1990;**259**:C279-C285

[82] Karim S, Adams DH, Lalor PF. Hepatic expression and cellular distribution of the glucose transporter family. World Journal of Gastroenterology. 2012;**18**:6771-6781

[83] Uldry M, Ibberson M, Hosokawa M, Thorens B. GLUT2 is a high affinity glucosamine transporter. FEBS Letters. 2002;**524**:199-203

[84] Bilir BM, Gong TW, Kwasiborski V, Shen CS, Fillmore CS, Berkowitz CM, et al. Novel control of the position-dependent expression of genes in hepatocytes. The GLUT-1 transporter. The Journal of Biological Chemistry. 1993;**268**:19776-19784

[85] Simpson IA, Appel NM, Hokari M, Oki J, Holman GD, Maher F. Blood-brain barrier glucose transporter: Effects of hypo- and hyperglycemia revisited. Journal of Neurochemistry. 1999;**72**:238-247

[86] Ebert BL, Firth JD, Ratcliffe PJ. Hypoxia and mitochondrial inhibitors regulate expression of glucose transporter-1 via distinct Cis-acting sequences. The Journal of Biological Chemistry. 1995;**270**:29083-29089

[87] Ng S, March S, Galstian A, Hanson K, Carvalho T, Mota MM, et al. Hypoxia promotes liver-stage malaria infection in primary human hepatocytes in vitro. Disease Models & Mechanisms. 2014;**7**:215-224

[88] Chen C, Pore N, Behrooz A, Ismail-Beigi F, Maity A. Regulation of glut1 mRNA by hypoxia-inducible factor-1. Interaction between H-ras and hypoxia. The Journal of Biological Chemistry. 2001;**276**:9519-9525

[89] Koseoglu MH, Beigi FI. Mechanism of stimulation of glucose transport in response to inhibition of oxidative phosphorylation: Analysis with myc-tagged Glut1. Molecular and Cellular Biochemistry. 1999;**194**:109-116

[90] Barnes K, Ingram JC, Porras OH, Barros LF, Hudson ER, Fryer LG. Activation of GLUT1 by metabolic and osmotic stress: Potential involvement of AMP-activated protein kinase (AMPK). Journal of Cell Science. 2002;**115**:2433-2442

[91] Egert S, Nguyen N, Schwaiger M. Myocardial glucose transporter GLUT1: Translocation induced by insulin and ischemia. Journal of Molecular and Cellular Cardiology. 1999;**31**:1337-1344

[92] Perrini S, Natalicchio A, Laviola L, Belsanti G, Montrone C, Cignarelli A. Dehydroepiandrosterone stimulates glucose uptake in human and murine adipocytes by inducing GLUT1 and GLUT4 translocation to the plasma membrane. Diabetes. 2004;**53**:41-52

[93] Abliz A, Deng W, Sun R, Guo W, Zhao L, Wang W. Wortmannin, PI3K/Akt signaling pathway inhibitor, attenuates thyroid injury associated with severe acute pancreatitis in rats. International Journal of Clinical and Experimental Pathology. 2015; **8**(11):13821-13833

[94] Lee EE, Ma J, Sacharidou A, Mi W, Salato VK, Nguyen N. A protein kinase C phosphorylation motif in GLUT1 affects glucose transport and is mutated in GLUT1 deficiency syndrome. Molecular and Cellular Biochemistry. 2015;**58**:845-853

[95] Pagliassotti MJ, Cherrington AD. Regulation of net hepatic glucose uptake in vivo. Annual Review of Physiology. 1992;**54**:847-860

[96] Danquah I, Bedu-Addo G, Mockenhaupt FP. Type 2 diabetes mellitus and increased risk for malaria infection. Emerging Infectious Diseases. 2010;**16**:1601-1604

[97] Wild S, Roglic G, Green A, Sicree R, King H. Global prevalence of diabetes: Estimates for the year 2000 and projections for 2030. Diabetes Care. 2004;**27**:1047-1053

[98] Raghunath P. Impact of type 2 diabetes mellitus on the incidence of malaria. Journal of Infection and Public Health. 2017;**10**:357-358. DOI: 10.1016/j.jiph.2016.08.013

[99] Ferguson MAJ, Brimacombe JS, Brown JR, Crossman A, Dix A, Field RA, et al. The GPI biosynthetic pathway as a therapeutic target for African sleeping sickness. Biochimica et Biophysica Acta. 1999;**1455**:327-340

[100] Miller LH, Roberts T, Shahabuddin M, M-C. TF. Analysis of sequence diversity in the *Plasmodium falciparum* merozoite surface protein-1 (MSP-1). Molecular and Biochemical Parasitology. 1993;**59**:1-14

[101] Naik RS, Davidson EA, Gowda DC. Developmental stage-specific biosynthesis of gly-cosylphosphatidylinositol anchors in intraerythrocytic *Plasmodium falciparum* and its inhibition in a novel manner by mannosamine. The Journal of Biological Chemistry. 2000;**275**:24506-24511

[102] Schofield L, Hackett F. Signal transduction in host cells by a glycosylphosphatidylinosi-tol toxin of malaria parasites. The Journal of Experimental Medicine. 1993;**1**(1):145-153

[103] Naik RS, Branch OH, Woods AS, Vijaykumar M, Perkins GJ, Nahlen BL, et al. Glycosyl-phosphatidylinositol anchors of *Plasmodium falciparum*: Molecular characterization and naturally elicited antibody response that may provide immunity to malaria pathogen-esis. Journal of Experimental Medicine. 2000;**192**(11):1563-1575

[104] Gowda DC. Structure and activity of glycosylphosphatidylinositol anchors of *Plasmodium falciparum*. Clinical Microbiology and Infection. 2002;**9**:983-990

[105] Taylor K, Bate CAW, Carr RE, Butcher GA, Taverne J, Playfair JHL. Phospholipid-containing toxic malaria antigens induce hypoglycaemia. Clinical and Experimental Immunology. 1992;**90**:1-5

[106] Caro HN, Sheikh NA, Taverne J, Playfair JHL, Rademacher TW. Structural similarities among malaria toxins, insulin second messengers, and bacterial endotoxin. Infection and Immunity. 1996;**64**(8):3438-3441 0019-9567/96/$04.0010

[107] Saliba KJ, Kirk K. pH regulation in the intracellular malaria parasite, *Plasmodium falciparum*. H(+) extrusion via a v-type h(+)-atpase. The Journal of Biological Chemistry. 1999;**274**:33213-33219

[108] Allen RJ, Kirk K. The membrane potential of the intraerythrocytic malaria parasite *Plasmodium falciparum*. The Journal of Biological Chemistry. 2004;**279**:11264-11272

[109] Slavic K, Krishna S, Derbyshire ET, Staines HM. Plasmodial sugar transporters as anti-malarial drug targets and comparisons with other protozoa. Malaria Journal. 2011;**10**:165

[110] Olszewski KL, Mather MW, Morrisey JM, Garcia BA, Vaidya AB, Rabinowitz JD, et al. Branched tricarboxylic acid metabolism in *Plasmodium falciparum*. Nature. 2010;**466**:774-778

[111] Manolescu AR, Witkowska K, Kinnaird A, Cessford T, Cheeseman C. Facilitated hexose transporters: New perspectives on form and function. Physiology (Bethesda). 2007;**22**:234-240

[112] Desai SA, Rosenberg RL. Pore size of the malaria parasite's nutrient channel. Proceedings of the National Academy of Sciences of the United States of America. 1997;**94**:2045-2049

[113] Woodrow CJ, Penny JI, Krishna S. Intraerythrocytic *Plasmodium falciparum* expresses a high affinity facilitative hexose transporter. The Journal of Biological Chemistry. 1999;**274**:7272-7277

[114] Kirk K, Horner HA, Elford BC, Ellory JC, Newbold CI. Transport of diverse substrates into malaria-infected erythrocytes via a pathway showing functional characteristics of a chloride channel. The Journal of Biological Chemistry. 1994;**269**:3339-3347

[115] Davis TM, Looareesuwan S, Pukrittayakamee S, Levy JC, Nagachinta B, White NJ. Glucose turnover in severe *falciparumm* malaria. Metabolism: Clinical and Experimental. 1993;**42**:334-340

[116] Kern P, Hemmer CJ, Van Damme J, Gruss HJ, Dietrich M. Elevated tumor necrosis factor alpha and interleukin-6 serum levels as markers for complicated *Plasmodium falciparum* malaria. The American Journal of Medicine. 1989;**87**:139-143

[117] Corssmit EP, Romijn JA, Sauerwein HP. Regulation of glucose production with special attention to nonclassical regulatoryy mechanisms: A review. Metabolism. 2001;**50**:742-755

[118] Newton CRJC, Krishna S. Severe *falciparum* malaria in children: Current understanding of pathophysiology and supportive treatment. Pharmacology Therapeutics. 1998;**79**:1-53

[119] Pukrittayakamee S, Krishna S, Ter Kuile F, Wilaiwan O, Williamson DH, White NJ. Alanine metabolism in acute falciparumm malaria. Tropical Medicine & International Health. 2002;**7**:911-918

[120] White NJ, Warrell DA, Chanthavanich P. Severe hypoglycemia and hyperinsulinemia in *falciparum* malaria. The New England Journal of Medicine. 1983;**309**:61-66

[121] White NJ, Miller KD, Marsh K. Hypoglycaemia in African children with severe malaria. Lancet. 1987;**1**:708-711

[122] Taylor TE, Molyneux ME, Wirima JJ, Alex Fletcher K, Morris K. Blood glucose levels in Malawian children beforee and during the administration of intravenous quinine for severe *falciparum* malaria. The New England Journal of Medicine. 1988;**319**:1040-1047

[123] Stumvoll M, Perriello G, Meyer C, Gerich J. Role of glutamine in human carbohydrate metabolism in kidney and otherr tissues. Kidney International. 1999;**55**:778-792

[124] Cowan G, Planche T, Agbenyega T. Plasma glutamine levels and falciparum malaria. Transactions of the Royal Society of Tropical Medicine and Hygiene. 1999;**93**:616-618

[125] Pukrittayakamee S, White NJ, Davis TM. Glycerol metabolism in severe *falciparum* malaria. Metabolism. 1994;**43**:887-892

[126] Corssmit EP, Romijn JA, Endert E, Sauerwein HP. Indomethacin stimulates basal glucose production in humans without changes in concentrations of glucoregulatory hormones. Clinical Science (Colch). 1993;**85**:679-685

[127] Keller CC, Davenport GC, Dickman KR, Hittner JB, Kaplan SS, Weinberg JB, et al. Suppression of prostaglandin E2 by malaria parasite products and antipyretics promotes overproduction of tumor necrosis factor-a association with the pathogenesis of childhood malarial anemia. The Journal of Infectious Diseases. 2006;**193**:1384-1393

[128] WHO. Communicable Diseases Cluster. Severe *falciparum* malaria. Transactions of the Royal Society of Tropical Medicine and Hygiene. 2000;**94**(Suppl 1):S1-90. PMID: 11103309

[129] Pukrittayakamee S, White NJ, Davis TM. Hepatic blood flow and metabolism in severe *falciparum* malaria: Clearance of intravenously administered galactose. Clinical Science (Colch). 1992;**82**:63-70

[130] Molyneux ME, Looareesuwan S, Menzies IS. Reduced hepatic blood flow and intestinal malabsorption in severe *falciparum* malaria. The American Journal of Tropical Medicine and Hygiene. 1989;**40**:470-476

[131] Onongbu IC, Onyeneke EC. Plasma lipid changes in human malaria. Annals of Tropical Medicine and Parasitology. 1983;**34**:193-196

[132] Davis TME, Pukrittayakamee S, Supanaranond W. Glucose metabolism in quinine-treated patients with uncomplicatedd *falciparum* malaria. Clinical Endocrinology. 1990;**33**:739-749

[133] Kawo NG, Msengi AE, Swai AB, Chuwa LM, Alberti KG, McLarty DG. Specificity of hypoglycaemia for cerebral malariaa in children. Lancet. 1990;**336**:454-547

[134] Taylor K, Carr R, Playfair JH, Saggerson ED. Malarial toxic antigens synergistically enhance insulin signalling. FFSS Letters. 1992;**311**:23M

[135] Visser BJ, Wieten RW, Nagel IM, Grobusch MP. Serum lipids and lipoproteins in malaria-A systematic review and meta-analysis. Malaria Journal. 2013;**12**:442

[136] Chu C, Sherck SM, K I. Effects of free fatty acids on hepatic glycogenosis and gluco-neogenesis in consciouss dogs. American Journal of Physiology. Endocrinology and Metabolism. 2002;**282**:E402-E411

[137] Stingl H, Krssak M, M K. Lipid-dependent control of hepatic glycogen stores in healthy humans. Diabetologia. 2001;**44**:48-54

[138] Boden G, Chen X, Capulong E, Mozzoli M. Effects of free fatty acids on gluconeogenesis and autoregulation of glucosee production in type 2 diabetes. Diabetes. 2001;**50**:810-816

[139] Roden M, Stingl H, Chandramouli V e a. Effects of free fatty acid elevation on postab-sorptive endogenous glucosee production and gluconeogenesis in humans. Diabetes. 2000;**49**:701-707

[140] Clore JN, Glickman PS, Nestler JE, Blackard WG. In vivo evidence for hepatic auto-regulation during FFA stimulated gluconeogenesis in normal humans. The American Journal of Physiology. 1991;**261**:E425-E429

[141] Lam TKT, Carpentier A, Lewis GF, Werve G, Fantus IG, Giacca A. Mechanisms of the free fatty acid-induced increase in hepatic glucose production. American Journal of Physiology. Endocrinology and Metabolism. 2003;**284**:E863-E873

[142] Taylor SM, Molyneux ME, Simel DL, Meshnick SR, Juliano JJ. Does this patient have malaria? Journal of the American Medical Association. 2010;**304**(18):2048-2056

[143] Chianura L, Errante IC, Travi G, Rossotti R, Puoti M. Hyperglycemia in severe falci-parum malaria: A case report. Case Reports in Critical Care (Hindawi Publish Corp). 2012;**2012**:3. DOI: 10.1155/2012/312458

[144] Zaki SA, Shanbag P. Atypical manifestations of malaria. Research and Reports in Tropical Medicine. 2011;**2**:9-22

[145] van Thien H, Ackermans MT, Dekker E. Glucose production and gluconeogenesis in adults with cerebral malaria. QJM: An International Journal of Medicine. 2001;**94**(12):709-715

[146] Dass R, Barman H, Duwarah SG, Deka NM, Jain P, Choudhury V. Unusual presentations of malaria in children: An experience from a tertiary care centre in North East India. Indian Journal of Pediatrics. 2010;**77**(6):655-660

[147] Clark IA, Budd AC, Alleva LM, Cowden WB. Human malarial disease: A consequence of inflammatory cytokine release. Malaria Journal. 2006;**5**:85. DOI: 10.1186/1475-2875-5-85

[148] Ramachandran V, Saravanan R. Efcacy of asiatic acid, a pentacyclic triterpene on attenuating the key enzymes activities of carbohydrate metabolism in streptozotoc ininduced diabetic rats. Phytomedicine. 2013;**20**:230-236

[149] Asamoah KA, Robb DA, Furman BL. Chronic chloroquine treatment enhances insulin release in rats. Diabetes Research and Clinical Practice. 1990;**9**:273-278

[150] Baker RG, Hayden MS. NF-kB, infammation, and metabolic disease. Cell Metabolism. 2011;**15**:11-22

[151] Grau GE, Fajardo LF, Piquet P-F, Allet B, Lambert P-H. Tumor necrosis factor (cachectin) as an essential mediator in murine cerebral malaria. Science. 1987;**237**:1210-1212

[152] Coxon RE, Fekade D, Knox K, Hussein K, Melka A. The efect of antibody against TNF alpha on cytokine response in Jarisch-Herxheimer reactions of louse-borne relapsing fever. The Quarterly Journal of Medicine. 1997;**90**:213-221

[153] Ramachandran V, Saravanan R, Senthilraja P. Antidiabetic and antihyperlipidemic activity of asiatic acid in diabetic rats, role of HMG CoA: In vivo and in silico approaches. Phytomedicine. 2014;**21**:225-232

[154] Chulman JL, Carleton JL, Whitney G, Whitehorn JC. Efect of glucagon on food intake and body weight in man. Journal of Applied Physiology. 1975;**11**:419-421

[155] Dabadghao VS, Singh VB, Sharma D, Meena BL. A study of serum lactate level in malaria and its correlation with severity of disease. International Journal of Advanced Medical and Health Research. 2015;**2**:28-32

Prevalence and Intensity of Intestinal Parasites and Malaria in Pregnant Women at Abobo District in Abidjan, Côte d'Ivoire

Gaoussou Coulibaly, Kouassi Patrick Yao,
Mathurin Koffi, Bernardin Ahouty Ahouty,
Laurent Kouassi Louhourignon, Monsan N'Cho and
Eliézer Kouakou N'Goran

Additional information is available at the end of the chapter

http://dx.doi.org/10.5772/intechopen.79699

Abstract

A prospective study was carried out from 2010 to 2012 at the Hôpital Général d'Abobo (HGA) in Abidjan, in order to determine the impact of infectious and parasitic diseases on child cognitive development. Blood samples were examined by means of drop thick and blood smear, as for stool by direct examination and concentration by formalin-ether method. We evaluated the prevalence and the parasite load of malaria and gastrointestinal parasites and then investigated the risk factors for these disorders. Overall, 331 pregnant women in the last trimester of their pregnancy were enrolled. The plasmodic index was 3.9% with an infestation specific rate for *P. falciparum* of 100%. Concerning digestive protozoa, it has been observed 71.3% of nonpathogenic, against 9.7% of pathogens, either an overall prevalence of 51.4% of digestive parasites. The calculated average parasitic loads revealed 3089.2 tpz/µl of blood (95% CI, 591.1–5587.3) for malaria, 6.5 eggs per gram of stool (95% CI, 0.4–13.4) for intestinal helminths, and one (1) parasite by microscopic field for protozoa (common infestation). It has been shown that the occurrence of malaria has been linked to the nonuse of impregnated mosquito nets ($\chi^2 = 0.012$, p = 0.018) to age. No link could be established between the presence of digestive parasites and the age of pregnant women or socioeconomic conditions (level of education, profession, type of toilet). Malaria is less common in pregnant women, while the rate of digestive parasites remains high.

Keywords: Abidjan, Côte d'Ivoire, intestinal parasites, malaria, pregnant women

1. Introduction

Intestinal parasitosis and malaria remain the most important diseases in sub-Saharan Africa [1, 2]. With hundreds of millions of sick people every year and about three million deaths per year, intestinal parasites and malaria remain the most important diseases in sub-Saharan Africa and mainly affect children and pregnant women [3, 4].

In pregnant women, these parasitic infections cause maternity accidents such as premature births, maternal-fetal death, and malformations [5–7].

In Côte d'Ivoire, malaria is the main cause of morbidity (40%) and mortality (10%) in the general population. Children under 5 years and pregnant women are the most affected. In addition to malaria, Côte d'Ivoire is facing other diseases such as intestinal parasitosis.

Long rural the tropical countries are confronted with the urban growth, with the biggest upheavals of the lifestyles of its history. Urbanization rate increased from 27.3% in 1975 to 49% in 2000 according to the United Nations estimates [8]. This represents an increase of about 1.3 billion people. Cities on the African continent are currently experiencing the strongest growth. The urbanization rate, which was only 13.2% in 1950, exceeded 37% in 2000, i.e., 270 million more urban dwellers [9]. This was the case for the city of Abidjan, the economic capital of Côte d'Ivoire, and more precisely in the municipality of Abobo. The urbanization of this town, which began in the 1970s, is so fast that nowadays Abobo already has more than one million inhabitants. However, infrastructure development has not kept pace with these rapid changes. In this context, precarious housing areas focus on pathologies linked to promiscuity, insalubrity, lack of drinking water supply, and/or poverty; these diseases are intestinal parasitosis and malaria [10, 11]. Moreover, it must be noted that few studies have been carried out on these parasites and particularly on pregnant women in this municipality. As part of a research project on the impact of infectious and parasitic diseases on the physical and mental development of children, pregnant women were followed up. The work consisted of evaluating the prevalence, parasite load of malaria, and digestive parasites and then determining risk factors of these parasitic infections in pregnant women in Abobo district in Abidjan.

2. Materials and methods

2.1. Study area and population

Our prospective study, which took place from May 2010 to June 2012 at the General Hospital of Abobo (GHA) in Abidjan, involved 331 pregnant women recruited in the last quarter of pregnancy; these future mothers all provided informed consent before being included in the study. They were aged 18–46 years. The mothers were recruited during antenatal clinic visits by gynecologists. Detailed explanations of the study were given by them in local languages if necessary.

The fact sheets on the socioeconomic status and study of risk factors have been met by community health workers (CHWs) in an interview with the mother following the signing of informed consent. It includes information on factors favoring the transmission of these parasites, namely, age, type of neighborhood, level of education, occupation, type of toilet, and use or not of impregnated mosquito nets.

2.2. Laboratory procedures: sample collection and parasitological analyzes

A blood sample of 5 ml was taken from patients by nurses, in a labeled EDTA tube (patient ID number) by venipuncture in the antecubital fossa, after disinfection of the sampling region by ethyl alcohol. Blood samples were stained in a solution of 10% Giemsa and microscopic reading of immersion oil at a magnification of 100. In the positive case, the parasitic identification was carried out on thin film, and parasite densities were evaluated from the thick drop of 200 or 500 leukocytes. Individual values obtained for parasitemia were finally reduced to microliter (1 μl) of blood on the basis of 8000 leucocytes by taking the product of the number of parasites obtained by 40 or 16, respectively, for 200 or 500 erythrocytes [12, 13].

A box for the stool sample was given to the mothers, and they were asked to return the next morning at the hospital with the boxes containing feces. The stools collected in the morning were labeled with the patient ID and were the subject of a direct microscopic examination between slide and cover glass. In addition, 1–1.5 g of stool was placed into a falcon tube containing 10 ml of sodium acetate–acetic acid formalin (SAF) solution, broken and homogenize with a wooden spatula and vigorously shaken. Within 1 month of stool collection, the SAF-fixed samples were subjected to an ether concentration method [14]; the SAF-fixed stool samples were re-suspended and filtered through medical gauze placed in a plastic funnel into a centrifuge tube. The first centrifugation is made at 2000 towers/min for 1 min. After centrifugation, the supernatant was discarded, and 7 ml of 0.9% NaCl plus 2–3 ml of ether was added to the remaining pellet. After shaking for 10–30 s, the tube and its content were centrifuged for 4–5 min at the same speed. Finally, from the four layers formed, the three top layers were discarded. The bottom layer, including the sediment, was examined under a microscope. With regard to the parasite load, the exact number of eggs of each species of helminth was marked; the presence of a species of protozoan was mentioned by a positive (+) sign. The number of + ranges from 1 to 3 depending on the intensity of the parasite. Indeed, 1+ corresponds to 1–5 parasites per analyzed microscopic slide, 2+ 1 parasite per microscopic field, and 3+ more than 1 parasite per microscopic field.

2.3. Statistical analysis

MS Excel software was used for entering data collected (parasitological data and those fact sheets) and perform figures.

Descriptive analysis was done to describe the data as counts, percentages, averages, using tables and figures. Statistical tests were carried out with the Stata software 11.0.

The chi-square test (χ^2) allowed us to appreciate the link between the occurrence of malaria and/or helminth infections and exposure factors (age, use of non-treated nets, socioeconomic conditions). The value of the probability (p) showed the degree of significance of the links at the 0.05 level. The Fisher exact test was used for small numbers (more than 5% of the theoretical frequencies less than 5).

2.4. Ethical considerations

The study conditions have been reviewed and approved by the National Ethics and Research Committee of Côte d'Ivoire (N ° 4169/MSHP). Detailed explanations of the study were given to mothers in local languages, if necessary. The participation was voluntary. When the mother consented, she signed or affixed a fingerprint on the informed consent sheet.

3. Results

3.1. Characteristics of study population

The study included 331 pregnant women from 13 neighborhoods in Abobo commune. The average age was 28.9 years old. The largest group of women was between 28 and 32 years old (31.7%) (**Figure 1**).

After the blood and stool examinations, 157 (47.4%) women presented no parasite. Four (4) women (1.2%) presented plasmodium, 161 (48.6%) digestive parasites, and nine (9) (2.7%) both parasites (**Table 1**).

3.2. Prevalence, parasite density, and risk factors of malaria

In total 13 women presented a positive thick smear of *Plasmodium* sp., with a parasite rate of 3.9%. Parasite mean of *Plasmodium falciparum* is 3089.2 trophozoïtes/µl of blood with a minimum of 360 trophozoïtes/µl and maximum of 13,400 trophozoïtes/µl. The highest prevalence (12.5%, 2/16) was recorded with the age group of 38 years and older and the lowest (1.2%, 1/83) with that of 23–27 years. The differences in prevalence observed between age groups are not statistically significant (x^2 = 5.11, p = 0.276). Infestation of *P. falciparum* is not age-related. Women not using treated nets are much more infested (6% 12/200) than those using insecticide (0.8%, 1/131). The parasitic porting is influenced by the use of treated mosquito nets (x^2 = 0.012, p = 0.018). Women not using bed nets are the most vulnerable to malaria (**Table 2**).

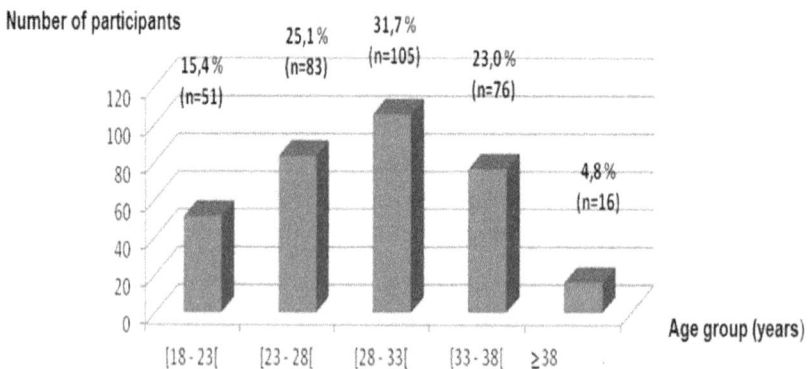

Figure 1. Distribution of population according to age.

Blood tests	Coprological analyzes		Total
	Negative digestive parasite	Positive digestive parasite	
Negative thick drop/blood smear	157 (47.4%)	161 (48.6%)	318 (96.1%)
Positive thick drop/blood smear	4 (1.2%)	9 (2.7%)	13 (3.9%)
Total	161 (48.6%)	170 (51.4%)	331 (100%)

Table 1. Distribution of participants according to the results of blood tests and stool.

	Using of treated mosquito nets		χ^2	p
	Oui	Non		
Number of participants	131	200		
Infected	1	12		
Prevalence (%)	0.8	3.9	0.012	0.018

Table 2. Prevalence of malaria according to the use or non-use of insecticide-treated bed nets.

Parasites species	Infected	Prevalence (%)
Protozoa		
Entamoeba coli	104	31.4
Endolimax nana	56	16.9
Blastocystis hominis	38	11.3
Entamoeba histolytica/dispar	23	7
Iodamoeba butschlii	15	4.5
Entamoeba hartmanni	12	3.6
Chilomastix mesnili	11	3.3
Giardia lamblia	9	2.7
Helminths		
Schistosoma mansoni	9	2.7
Trichuris trichiura	4	1.2
Ascaris lumbricoïdes	1	0.3

Table 3. Prevalence of intestinal parasites species.

3.3. Prevalence, infection intensities, and risk factors of intestinal parasites

After stool examinations, eight (8) species of intestinal protozoa belonging to six (6) different kinds were diagnosed in Abobo. These are *Entamoeba histolytica/dispar*, *Giardia lamblia*,

Endolimax nana, Entamoeba coli, Iodamoeba butschlii, Chilomastix mesnili, Entamoeba hartmanni, and *Blastocystis hominis.* The term *"Entamoeba histolytica/dispar"* was used because the method used for stool examinations did not allow to distinguish the species *Entamoeba histolytica* and *Entamoeba dispar.*

In addition to these protozoa, three species of helminths were observed: *Schistosoma mansoni, Trichuris trichiura,* and *Ascaris lumbricoides.* Of the 331 women screened, 170 were carriers of digestive parasites, with an overall prevalence of 51.4%. The prevalence of species of digestive parasites (pathogenic and nonpathogenic protozoa of digestive and intestinal helminths) is presented in **Table 3**. With protozoa, the highest prevalence was observed with *Entamoeba coli* (31.4%, 104/331) and *Endolimax nana* (16.9%, 56/331). Concerning intestinal helminths, in the three species, *Schistosoma mansoni* was the most abundant with a prevalence of 2.7%. In terms of parasite load protozoa, the trend observed in our study was 2+, namely, 1 parasite per microscope field, the latter being described as frequent infestation. As regards the helminths, the average worm burden was 7.8 eggs/gram of feces. The most infested age group is that of 23–27 years (59%, 49/83), while the least infested was that of 18–22 years (45.1%, 23/51). Age had no significant association with gastrointestinal parasites ($\chi^2 = 3.77$, p = 0.438). These parasites infest all age groups. No significant binding was recorded between the digestive parasites and level of schooling ($\chi^2 = 6.88$, p = 0.76), occupation ($\chi^2 = 2.66$, p = 0.103) (Table 5), and the type of toilets ($\chi^2 = 1.57$, p = 0.456). The occurrence of intestinal parasites is not related to the socioeconomic conditions.

4. Discussion

We examined 331 pregnant women of which 13 showed positive thick smear, with a parasite rate of 3.9%. Menan et al. [15] had reported in 1996 had a higher prevalence of 18.8% among the population of Abidjan. Our low rate could be explained by the fact that pregnant women receive intermittent preventive treatment (IPT) with sulfadoxine-pyrimethamine (SP) against malaria during pregnancy.

P. falciparum has been the only species identified during our work with a specific index of 100%. During these works in Côte d'Ivoire [16, 17], all cases of infection were also due to *P. falciparum.* By cons, it was highlighted at Taï southwestern Côte d'Ivoire the coexistence of *P. falciparum, P. malariae,* and *P. ovale* with specific rates of 84, 14, and 2% [18]. These studies highlight the prevalence of *P. falciparum* in Côte d'Ivoire (80–97% of infections) [19, 20].

The minimum parasitemia is 360 tpz/µl and the maximum 13,400 tpz/µl of blood. The average parasite density was 3089.2 tpz/µl of blood during the study. Our low parasite density could be explained by the fact that we have a gradual reduction in parasite densities with age [19]. Furthermore, it was suggested that the gradual decline in parasite densities with age is associated with the acquisition of immunity [21].

Our study revealed that the incidence of malaria is not related to age of the pregnant woman. This observation is similar to that of Menan et al. [15] in 1996 at the Abidjan population.

It appears from our study that there is a link between malaria and the use or non-treated nets. Women using treated nets are much less infested than those not using bed nets. Furthermore, the use of treated nets is a means of prevention against malaria [22].

During our study, slightly more than half of pregnant women were carriers of digestive parasites (pathogenic and nonpathogenic protozoa and intestinal helminths), with a rate of 51.4%. This rate is similar to that reported in pregnant women from Abidjan and its suburbs (53.6%) [23]. This demonstrates that the digestive parasites remain in pregnant women in Abidjan and maintain their level of infestation. The most common species of protozoa in our study area are nonpathogenic species *E. coli* (31.4%) and *E. nana* (16.9%). This same predominance was observed in 1993 among pregnant women in Abidjan [23]. The both pathogenic species of digestive protozoans (*E. histolytica/dispar*, *G. lamblia*) have a cumulative rate of 9.7%, which is substantially equal to that commonly found in children of school age (9.1%) [24], which demonstrated that this pathogenic protozoa infest either the mothers or the children in our study area.

Overall, helminths are not often found in our study. The predominant species is *Schistosoma mansoni* (2.7%), followed by *Trichuris trichiura* (1.2%) and *Ascaris lumbricoides* (0.3%). The prevalence of *Schistosoma mansoni* (2.72%) is in the prevalence interval (0.1–7.5%) indicated in Ivorian urban areas [25]. Prevalence close to that obtained in this study, namely, 3.1 and 3.9%, has been reported in Abidjan [26, 27]. This rate is higher than that observed (0.8%) among school age children in Abidjan [28]. This prevalence is low compared to those found in Moapé (Adzopé) (75%) [29] and Azaguié (Agboville) (88%) [30]. It must be emphasized that Agboville and Adzopé are schistosomiasis endemic areas [29, 31]. *Trichuris trichiura* was found at a rate of 1.2%. This rate is superimposed on that of Raso et al. [30] in 2005 in Man (1.3%). A much higher rate than ours was obtained in Agboville (15%), in a study in schools [32]. Furthermore, it is clear that the prevalence of trichuriasis is significantly higher than in the forest zone savanna [25, 33]. However, our very low prevalence could be explained by the analysis technique (method of concentration by formalin-ether) used. The prevalence of *Ascaris lumbricoides* was 0.3%. In a survey in Toumodi, no cases of roundworm porting have been reported [34]. A prevalence of 31.2% of roundworm porting was noted in Bondoukou; they felt it was the most common parasite in north-western Côte d'Ivoire [35].

This situation of frequent infestation (one parasite per field) to protozoa may be explained by the fact that the clean Abobo has many shortcomings, namely, unhealthiness linked to the failure of systems' sewage and promoting fecal peril.

Regarding helminths, the low-average parasite burden (7.8 eggs/g of stool) could be the fact that we used direct examination and SAF technique for stool examination. These techniques are very sensitive for the detection of helminth species compared to the Kato-Katz technique. Furthermore, the technique of concentration by formalin-ether remains one of the most suited for the identification of intestinal protozoa techniques.

Our study reveals that the parasite carriage is not related to age. However, the age group most affected is that of 23–27 years (59%). This is consistent with that of N'Guemby and Le Bigot [36] in Libreville in Gabon which have found a high prevalence among participants from 21 to 31 years in 1981. This finding could be justified by the fact that this age range is very involved in the household.

Our study showed that there is no significant link between the species of digestive parasites and socioeconomic conditions (level of education, occupation, type of toilet). This same observation was made in adults residing in Bangkok, Thailand [37].

5. Conclusion

We noted a decrease in the rate of malaria in pregnant women compared with previous studies; the rate of digestive parasites remains high. These results appear in connection with the effectiveness of the policy against malaria despite the poor hygiene of these populations.

6. Summary

Intestinal parasitosis and malaria diseases, among others, remain the largest problem in sub-Saharan Africa; they mainly affect children (under 5 years) and pregnant women. Our study objective was to identify species of malarial and digestive parasites and to estimate the prevalence and intensity of infestation of these parasites and clarify the risk factors for these infections in pregnant women from the commune of Abobo. Our study was conducted at the General Hospital of Abobo (HGA) in Abidjan. This is a prospective study (2010–2012). Overall, 331 pregnant women in the last trimester of gestation, antenatal clinic goers, were recruited. They were aged 18–46 years. Blood samples were examined by thick film techniques and blood smears; stool samples were collected for direct examination, and method of concentration is formalin-ether. Intermittent treatment against malaria with sulfadoxine-pyrimethamine has contributed significantly to the reduction of malaria among pregnant women. The rate of digestive parasites remains high, indicating poor hygiene practice in these women.

Acknowledgements

We thank the Deutsche Forschungsgemeinschaft Germany (DFG) for the financing of this project. We are grateful to the director and the staff of Hôpital Général d'Abobo (Abidjan, Côte d'Ivoire) and community health workers (CHW) for their support and for facilitating the implementation of our study. We thank the pregnant women (mothers) for their enthusiastic participation.

Conflict of interest

There is no conflict of interest.

Author details

Gaoussou Coulibaly[1]*, Kouassi Patrick Yao[1], Mathurin Koffi[2], Bernardin Ahouty Ahouty[3],
Laurent Kouassi Louhourignon[1], Monsan N'Cho[4] and Eliézer Kouakou N'Goran[1]

*Address all correspondence to: gaoussoubrava@yahoo.fr

1 Laboratoire de Zoologie et Biologie Animale, Université Félix Houphouët-Boigny, UFR
Biosciences, Abidjan, Côte d'Ivoire

2 Laboratoire des Interactions Hôte-Microorganisme-Environnement et Evolution (LIHME),
Université Jean Lorougnon Guédé, UFR Environnement, Daloa, Côte d'Ivoire

3 Laboratoire de Génétique, Université Félix Houphouët-Boigny, UFR Biosciences,
Abidjan, Côte d'Ivoire

4 Centre de Recherche et de Lutte contre le Paludisme (CRLP), Institut National de Santé
Publique de Côte d'Ivoire, Abidjan, Côte d'Ivoire

References

[1] Greenwood B, Mutabingwa T. Malaria in 2002. Nature. 2002;**415**:670-672

[2] Dianou D, Poda JN, Savadogo LG, et al. Intestinal parasite in the Sourou hydroagricultural system zone of Burkina faso. VertigO. 2004;**5**:3-10

[3] WHO. Burden of disease in disability-adjusted life years (DALYs) by cause, sex and mortality stratum in who regions, estimates for 2000. Report 2001, annex table 3. Geneva: WHO-Health statistics and informations; 2001

[4] Bejon P, Tabitha WM, Brett L, et al. Helminth infection and eosinophilia and the risk of *Plasmodium falciparum* malaria in 1-to 6-year-old children in a malaria endemic area. PLoS Neglected Tropical Diseases. 2008;**2**(2):164

[5] Van Heydan A. Intestinal Worms. Kinshasa: Ed Marketing; 1978. p. 80

[6] Bourée P, Leméteyer MF. Tropical Diseases and Pregnancy. Vol. 1 vol. Paris, France: Ed Pradel; 1990. 228 pp

[7] Bricaire, Gentilini M. Parasitosis and Pregnancy. Act Therap Internationale, Sanofi et Winthrop. 1993;**19**:10-11

[8] United Nations. Test estimation of the number of the men. Population. 2000;**1**:6

[9] UNICEF. Summary of Deworming Activities in West and Central Africa and joint WHO-UNICEF on Deworming. New York; 2006. p. 40

[10] Gentilini M. Parasitic diseases. In: Tropical Medicine. Paris: Flammarion Médecine-Sciences; 1995. pp. 159-173

[11] WHO. Treatment of Diarrhea. A Manuel for Physicians and Other Qualified Personnel. 4th rev. Geneva: World Health Organization; 2006. p. 43

[12] Henry MC, Rogier C, Nzeyimana L, et al. Inland valley rice production systems and malaria infection and disease in the savannah of Côte d'Ivoire. Tropical Medicine & International Health. 2003;**8**:449-458

[13] Iqbal J, Muneer A, Khalid N, et al. Performance of OptiMal test for malaria diagnosis among suspected malaria patients at the rural health centers. The American Journal of Tropical Medicine and Hygiene. 2003;**68**:624-628

[14] Utzinger J, Botero-Kleiven S, Castelli F, et al. Microscopic diagnosis of sodium acetate-acetic acid-formalin-fixed stool samples for helminths and intestinal protozoa: A comparison among European reference laboratories. Clinical Microbiology and Infection. 2008;**16**:267-273

[15] Menan EIH, Adou-Bryn KD, Mobio SP, et al. Total parasitological examinations of blood for malaria research at the Institut Pasteur de Côte d'Ivoire (I. P. C. I.). Médecine d'Afrique Noire. 1996;**43**(3):129-133

[16] Raso G, Utzinger J, Silué KD, et al. Disparities in parasitic infections, perceived ill-health and access to health care delivery structures among more and less poor school children of rural Côte d'Ivoire. Tropical Medicine & International Health. 2005;**11**:42-57

[17] Eholié SP, Ehui E, Adou-bryn K, et al. Severe malaria in Aboriginal in Abidjan (Côte d'Ivoire). Bulletin de la Société de Pathologie Exotique. 2004;**2551**:340-344

[18] Nzeyimana L, MC H, Dossou-Yovo J. Malaria epidemiology in the forest Southwestern of Côte d'Ivoire (Taï region). Bulletin de la Société de Pathologie Exotique. 2002;**95**(2):89-94

[19] Silué KD, Felger I, Utzinger J, et al. Prevalence, antigenic diversity and multiplicity of *Plasmodium falciparum* infection in school children in Central Côte d'Ivoire. Médecine Tropicale. 2006;**66**:137-142

[20] Yavo W, Ackra KN, Menan EIH. Comparative study of four biological diagnostic techniques used malaria in Côte d'Ivoire. Bulletin de la Société de Pathologie Exotique. 2002;**95**(4):238-240

[21] Smith T, Felger I, Tanner M, Beck H-P. Epidemiology of multiple Plasmodium falciparum infections. 11. Premunition in Plasmodium falciparum: insights from epidemiology of multiple infections. Transactions of the Royal Society of Tropical Medicine and Hygiene. 1999;**93**(Suppl. 1):59-64

[22] Koudou BG, Tano Y, Doumbia M, et al. Malaria transmission dynamics in Central Côte d'Ivoire: The influence of changing patterns of irrigated rice agriculture. Medical and Veterinary Entomology. 2005;**19**:27-37

[23] Penali LK, Broalet EY, Koné M. Helminth and protozoan infections in pregnant women in Côte d'Ivoire. Médecine d'Afrique Noire. 1993;**40**(5):353-356

[24] Konaté A. Support for carrying *Giardia intestinalis* cysts, *Entamoeba coli* and *Endolimax nana* by Metronidazole association and Diloxanide Furoate. The Pharma Abidjan. 2006; **1027**:108

[25] Doucet J, Assalé G. Epidemiology of intestinal helminths in Côte d'Ivoire. Médecine d'Afrique Noire. 1982;**29**(8-9):573-576

[26] Rouamba E, Menan EIH, Ouhon J, et al. Intestinal helminth infection: Results of five years of parasitic coprology at the Institut Pasteur de Cocody (Abidjan – Côte d'Ivoire). Médecine d'Afrique Noire. 1997;**44**(7):416-419

[27] Assalé G, Ferly-Therizol M, Koné M. Helminth and protozoan intestinal in Abidjan. Revue Médicale de Côte d'Ivoire. 1986;**75**:179-180

[28] Menan EIH, Nebavi NGF, Abjetey TAK, et al. Profile of helminthes among schoolchildren in Abidjan. Bulletin de la Société de Pathologie Exotique. 1997;**90**:51-54

[29] Nozais JP, Doucet J. The method of KATO: value compared with other methods of single stool examination in detecting intestinal helminths. Médecine d'Afrique Noire. 1976;**23**(numéro spécial):74-79

[30] Coulibaly TJ, Fürst T, Silué KD, et al. Intestinal parasitic infections in schoolchildren in different settings of Côte d'Ivoire: Effect of diagnostic approach and implications for control. Parasites & Vectors. 2012;**5**:135

[31] Guessand G, Koffi JK, Monges P. Intestinal helminths and public health. Médecine d'Afrique Noire. 1982;**29**(8-9):633-638

[32] Oga Agbaya SS, Yavo W, Menan EIH, et al. Intestinal helminths in schoolchildren: Preliminary results of the prospective study in Agboville in Southern Côte d'Ivoire. Cahier santé. 2004;**14**:143-147

[33] Nozais JP, Dunand J, Doucet J. Evaluation of the main intestinal parasites in 860 Ivoirian children from 13 villages. Médecine Tropicale. 1981;**41**:181-185

[34] Adou-Bryn D, Kouassi M, Brou J, et al. Prevalence of parasitosis to oral transmission among children in Toumodi (Côte d'Ivoire). Médecine d'Afrique Noire. 2001;**10**(48):394-398

[35] Penali LK, Adje E, Koné M, et al. Intestinal parasites in the region of Bondoukou (Côte d'Ivoire). Médecine d'Afrique Noire. 1989;**82**:60-64

[36] N'Guemby MC, Le Bigot P. Digestive parasites in Libreville. Bulletin Médical d'Owendo. 1981:37-39

[37] Pitisuttithum P, Migasena S, Juntra A. Socio-economic in Thaï. Adult residing in and around Bangkok metropolis. Journal of the Medical Association of Thailand. 1990; **73**(9):522-534

Chapter 5

Current Aspects in Trichinellosis

José Luis Muñoz-Carrillo, Claudia Maldonado-Tapia,
Argelia López-Luna, José Jesús Muñoz-Escobedo,
Juan Armando Flores-De La Torre and
Alejandra Moreno-García

Additional information is available at the end of the chapter

http://dx.doi.org/10.5772/intechopen.80372

Abstract

Currently, it is estimated that more than 11 million humans in the world are infected by helminth parasites of *Trichinella* species, mainly by *Trichinella spiralis* (*T. spiralis*), responsible for causing Trichinellosis disease in both animals and humans. Trichinellosis is a cosmopolitan parasitic zoonotic disease, which has direct relevance to human and animal health, because it presents a constant and important challenge to the host's immune system, especially through the intestinal tract. Currently, there is an intense investigation of new strategies in pharmacotherapy and immunotherapy against infection by *Trichinella spiralis*. In this chapter, we will present the most current aspects of biology, epidemiology, immunology, clinicopathology, pharmacotherapy and immunotherapy in Trichinellosis.

Keywords: Trichinellosis, immune response, pharmacotherapy, resiniferatoxin, immunotherapy

1. Introduction

Over 2 billion people are infected with helminth parasites worldwide [1, 2], making them one of the most prevalent infectious agents, responsible for many diseases in both animals and humans [3], thus being a public health problem throughout the world [4]. Research in these parasitic infections is of direct relevance to human and animal health [5], due to its capacity to cause great morbidity and socioeconomic loss [1]. In both humans and animals, helminth parasites establish chronic infections associated with significant downregulation of the immune response [6, 7], inducing a broad spectrum of pathological responses and clinical manifestations, which result in increased morbidity in affected individuals [1].

Trichinellosis is the parasitic disease caused by the parasitic helminth species of the genus *Trichinella* [8], which is a zoonotic parasitic disease, resulting from the consumption of meat from infected animals [9]. Currently, 12 species have been identified, which are classified into two clades: (1) the clade of the encapsulated species: *T. spiralis* (**Figure 1**), *T. native, T. britovi, T. nelsoni, T. murrelli* and *T. patagoniensis*, T6, T8 and T9 and (2) the clade of non-encapsulated species *T. pseudospiralis, T. papuae* and *T. zimbawensis* [11–13].

2. Epidemiological aspects of Trichinellosis

Trichinellosis is a parasitic disease, which is characterized by a wide range of hosts, including humans, mammals and birds, as well as a cosmopolitan disease because it has a wide geographical distribution [14–16]. Trichinellosis probably originated in wild animal populations of the Arctic and subarctic regions; later, it was extended to the animal populations of the temperate and tropical zones [17].

According to the World Health Organization (WHO) until the year 2009, there were more than 65,000 cases of Trichinellosis in the world, with more than 42 fatal cases [18] in the regions of Africa, South Asia, Europe [12, 19] and America, mainly United States, Mexico, Chile and Argentina [20], because of its high infectivity. However, it is estimated that currently 11 million humans in the world are infected by the *Trichinella* species, mainly by *T. spiralis* [18]. In 2014, Food and Agriculture Organization of the United Nations (FAO), together with the WHO, published a list of the top 10 food-borne parasites that affect the health of millions of people

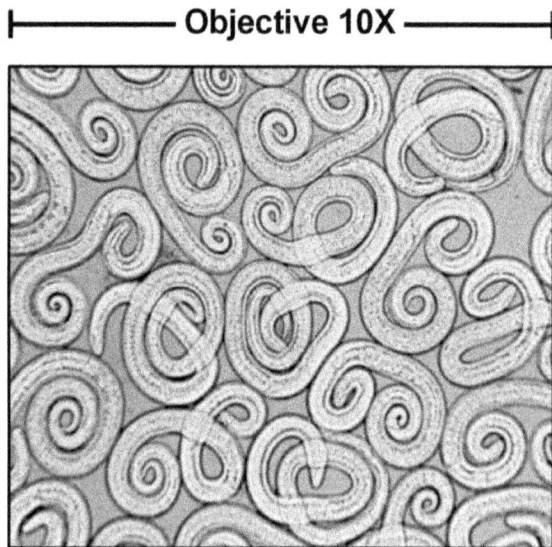

Figure 1. Infective larvae of *T. spiralis*. Photomicrograph of infective larvae of *T. spiralis*, from artificial digestion, observed at a 10× objective under the light optical microscope [10].

every year worldwide, infecting muscle tissues and organs and causing serious health problems. *T. spiralis* occupied the seventh place, below parasites of medical importance such as *Taenia solium* (*T. solium*), *Toxoplasma gondii* (*T. gondii*) and *Entamoeba histolytica* (*E. histolytica*); therefore, currently Trichinellosis remains a food-borne parasitic disease of great medical importance worldwide [21], and its impact and magnitude of the problem that this parasitic disease represents become evident only in the appearance of epidemic outbreaks [22].

In recent years, the reported rates of Trichinellosis in Mexico have been reduced to levels that are comparable to those of the United States. In fact, Canada now reports one of the highest rates in North America [23]. In Mexico, human Trichinellosis frequently occurs from the ingestion of raw or undercooked pork [9, 24]. In general, in Mexico, there is little knowledge of the disease, and in existing epidemiological studies by post-mortem histopathology of humans, prevalence of 50% has been observed, while in hospitals it is from 4 to 15% [25]. Since 1990 to date, more than 1122 cases of human Trichinellosis have been reported in at least 17 states of the country such as Aguascalientes, Chihuahua, Mexico City, Colima, Durango, State of Mexico, Guanajuato, Guerrero, Jalisco, Michoacán, Nuevo León, Oaxaca, Querétaro, San Luis Potosí, Veracruz and Zacatecas [25–27]. In Zacatecas, it has been considered as a zoonosis; since 1976, more than 100 cases have been reported in humans, pigs, dogs and domestic rats [28–30].

3. Biology of *Trichinella spiralis*

James Paget, a medical student at St. Bartholomew's Hospital in London, England, observed a parasite in the diaphragm muscle of a 51-year-old Italian patient who had died from tuberculosis. Subsequently, the British zoologist Richard Owen in 1835 studied portions of muscle tissue of the Paget case and gave it the name of *T. spiralis* [31]. The adult parasites of *T. spiralis* were discovered by Rudolf Virchow in 1859 and Friedrich Zenker in 1860, who finally recognized the clinical importance of the infection and concluded that humans become infected by eating raw meat infected with the parasite [32].

The epidemic of this zoonosis is very particular, since the "domestic" and "wild" cycles of the *T. spiralis* have been clearly studied. But between them is the synanthropic cycle. In the domestic cycle (**Figure 2**), the main transmission vector to humans is the pig, through the ingestion of meat infected with *T. spiralis*. In the wild cycle, *T. spiralis* is kept in the environment by predatory and scavenger animals and can enter the domestic cycle accidentally. While in the synanthropic cycle, animals such as rats, cats, dogs, foxes, mustelids, among others, act as transmission vectors for the different *Trichinella* genotypes involved in any of the two mentioned cycles [33].

The main characteristic of the epidemiology of *T. spiralis* is its obligatory transmission by ingestion of infected meat [34, 35]. When a host ingests meat infected with L1 of *T. spiralis* (*T. spiralis*-L1), the digestive juices of the stomach dissolve the collagen capsule [36], also called nurse cell (NC), releasing the *T. spiralis*-L1, which travel to the small intestine, where they invade the columnar epithelium [37], giving rise to the intestinal phase of the infection (**Figure 2**).

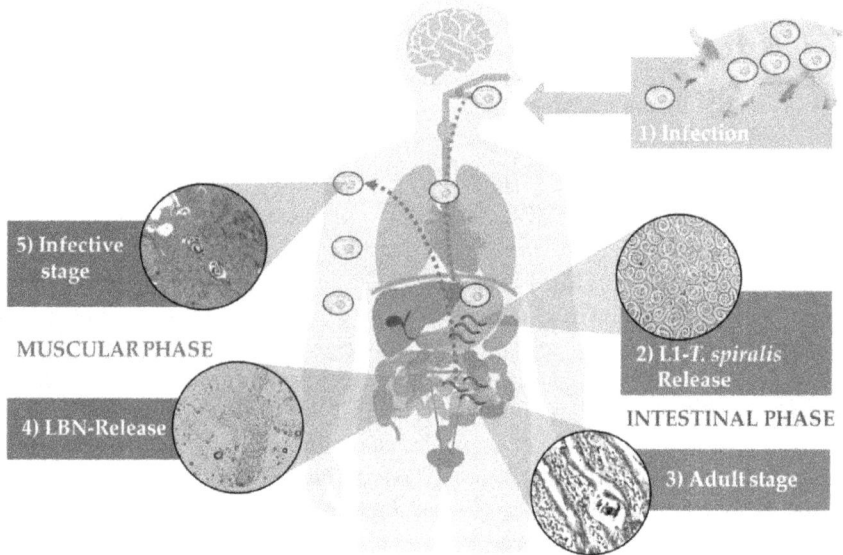

Figure 2. Life cycle of *Trichinella spiralis*. (1) Ingestion of meat infected with L1-*T. spiralis*. Intestinal phase: (2) Release of L1-*T. spiralis* in the stomach. (3) Migration of *T. spiralis*-L1 to the small intestine and maturation to female and male adult worms of *T. spiralis*. (4) Reproduction of adult worms of *T. spiralis* and release of newborn larvae (NBL) of *T. spiralis*. Muscle phase: (5) Migration of NBL *T. spiralis* and invasion of skeletal muscle cells to develop to infective stage of *T. spiralis* forming the complex nurse cell (NC) and L1-*T. spiralis*.

After 10–30 hours post-infection (pi), *T. spiralis*-L1 mature to female and male adult worms (AD). Approximately 7 days pi, copulation occurs between female and male AD. Embryogenesis lasts about 90 hours, since the newborn larvae (NBL) of *T. spiralis* are released [38, 39]. These NBL of *T. spiralis* possess a stylet in their oral cavity, which they use to internalize within the epithelial cells of the host [36], penetrating the submucosa of the small intestine, migrating mainly through the circulatory system to various organs and subsequently invading the musculoskeletal cells, causing tissue damage (**Figure 2**). Only the NBL of *T. spiralis* that invade the musculoskeletal cells can survive and grow [15], giving rise to the muscle phase of the infection. During the muscular phase (**Figure 2**), the NBL of *T. spiralis* are in the muscle fibers, destroying them partially, and begin a period of post-embryonic development, growing and developing exponentially [36, 38, 39]. Approximately at 15 days pi, the formation of NC is induced with a fusiform or elongated aspect, containing in its interior one or several L1-*T. spiralis*, forming the NC-L1 complex [40]. The NC formation process is a complex process and includes the cellular response of the infected muscle (from differentiation with a complete loss of the myofibrillar organization, re-entry and arrest of the cell cycle in G2/M) and the responses of the NC (cells undergo activation, proliferation, redifferentiation and fusion processes with each other or with the infected muscle cell). Since the satellite cell is a progenitor cell located within the capsule wall, a new cell can be continuously delivered from the myoblast, even if the present NC dies. This explains why CN seems intact and active for years despite intracellular parasitism. In this way, the parasites use the muscular mechanisms of cellular repair of the host to establish parasitism [41]. *T. spiralis* develops its infectious stage approximately between days 21 and 30 pi, and six months after infection, the deposit of calcium begins in the NC walls, calcifying in 1 year. L1-*T. spiralis* can be retained for several years, depending on the host species. L1-*T. spiralis* appears to be non-pathogenic for natural hosts except for humans [15, 42]. The main striated muscles where the L1-*T. spiralis* is implanted are the most active such as the diaphragm, masseters, intercostals, eye muscles, muscles of the tongue, and anterior and posterior extremities (**Figure 2**) [43, 44].

4. Clinical pathology of Trichinellosis

The severity of the clinical disease is strongly dependent and directly correlated with the number of L1-*T. spiralis* ingested, age, sex, invaded tissue, nutritional, hormonal and immune status. Likewise, the infection can give rise to a wide spectrum of clinical forms, from asymptomatic to mortality [14, 17, 45].

The clinical pathology of Trichinellosis can be divided based on the phases of the *T. spiralis* life cycle (**Figure 3**). Infections with low parasite burden can remain asymptomatic, while high parasite burden can cause gastroenteritis associated with diarrhea and abdominal pain, approximately 24–48 hours pi (acute phase of infection) [46]. The intestinal phase of Trichinellosis is clinically manifested by the presence of signs, symptoms and gastrointestinal disorders, such as malaise, mild transient diarrhea, nausea, vomiting, abdominal pain, chills and fever, due to the invasion of L1-*T. spiralis* and AD worms in the intestinal mucosa (**Figure 3**). These signs and symptoms usually persist from the first to the third week pi, depending on the dose of L1-*T. spiralis* and the severity of the disease. From 2 to 6 weeks pi, the intestinal phase is still present, but the signs and symptoms that correlate with the intestinal disease decrease and the signs and symptoms of the migration phase appear [14, 38, 42, 47].

During the migration of NBL of *T. spiralis*, which starts approximately 1 week pi and may last for several weeks [36], the first signs and symptoms to be clinically detected usually include myalgia, high fever, chills, a state like paralysis, periorbital and/or facial edema, conjunctivitis, pain, skin rashes, etc. (**Figure 3**) [14, 38, 42]. Other signs and symptoms are conjunctivitis including subconjunctival hemorrhages, headache, dry cough, petechial hemorrhages and painful movement disorder of the eye muscles. Some patients present urticaria, maculopapular rash and subungual hemorrhages, caused by vasculitis, the main pathological process of Trichinellosis [14]. Laboratory studies reveal a moderate increase in white blood cells (12,000–15,000 cells/mm^3), and circulating eosinophilia ranging from 5 to 50% [35, 45].

During the muscular phase of Trichinellosis, signs and symptoms such as myalgias, arthralgia, headache, periorbital and facial edema appear (**Figure 3**) [42]. The damage of the muscular cell stimulates the infiltration of inflammatory cells, mainly eosinophils. A correlation between levels of eosinophils and serum muscle enzymes, such as lactate dehydrogenase (LDH) and creatine phosphokinase (CPK), has been observed in patients with Trichinellosis, suggesting that muscle damage may be mediated indirectly by these activated granulocytes [14]. Thus, progressive eosinophilia is the most relevant clinical finding of the muscular phase of Trichinellosis [42]. The invasion of the diaphragm and accessory muscles of respiration by the parasite results in dyspnea [36]. In the chronic phase of the Trichinellosis after 4 weeks pi, a series of complications such as encephalitis, bronchopneumonia and sepsis arise. Chronic

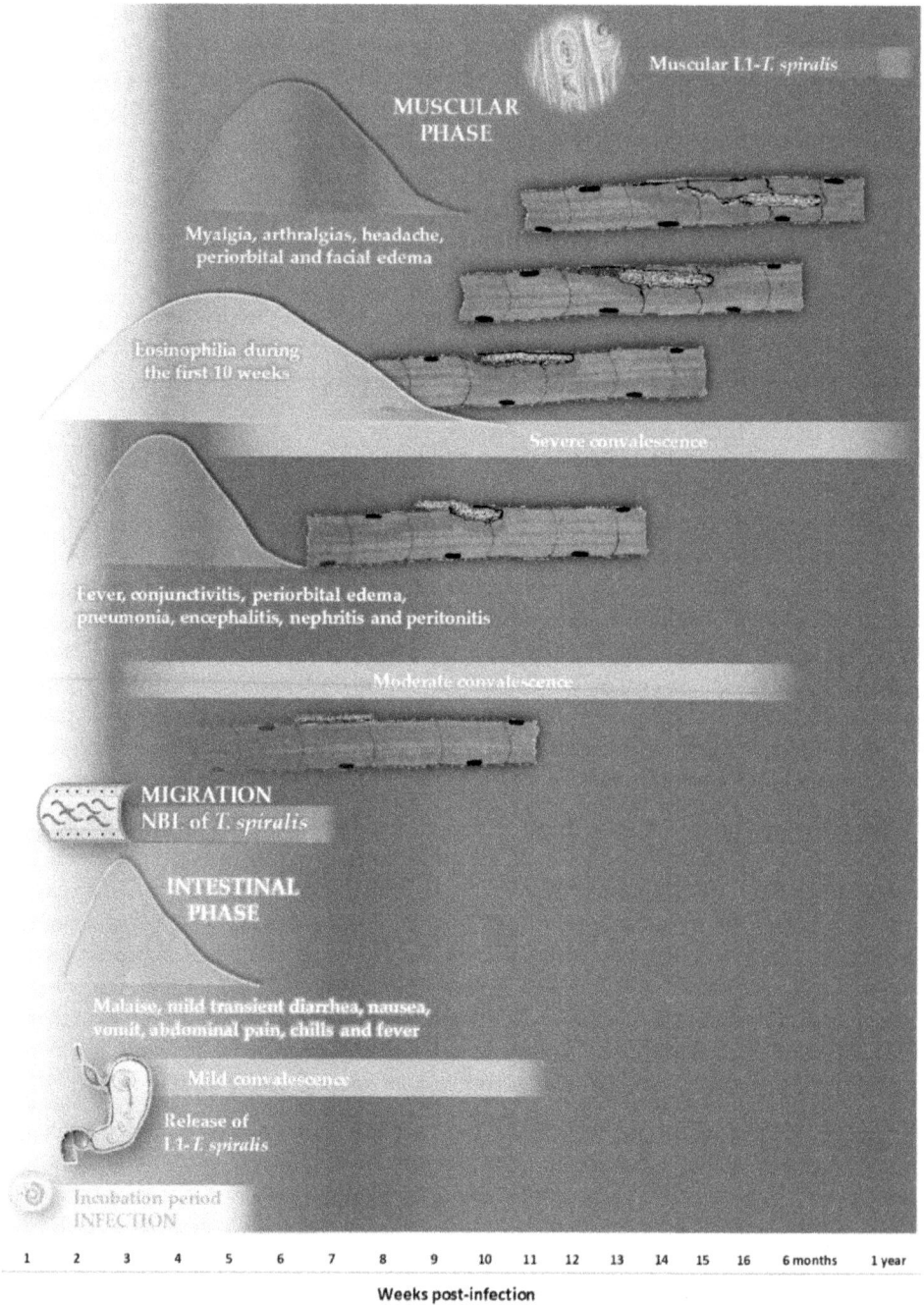

Figure 3. Clinical pathology of Trichinellosis. Main clinical signs and symptoms of Trichinellosis. Intestinal phase (green), migration phase (blue) and muscular phase (red). This figure was made by the authors based on the references cited in the text.

Trichinellosis can cause persistent tingling, numbness and excessive sweating, as well as deterioration of muscle strength and conjunctivitis, which can persist up to 10 years in people who had not been treated early in the acute phase of the infection [14].

5. Immune response against *Trichinella spiralis*

In each phase of the life cycle of *T. spiralis*, different antigenic components are produced, which directly influence the host's immune response [48] and are very useful in the diagnosis of Trichinellosis in both humans and animals. These antigens, *T. spiralis* larvae group (TSL)-1, are secreted and/or excreted by the L1-*T. spiralis* at the beginning of the intestinal phase and again in the muscular phase of the infection when the NC is formed [49–51]. The antigens TSL-1 are glycoproteins 43 [52–55], 53 [56–59] and 45 [60, 61] kDa, which are targets of antibodies that mediate humoral immunity against *T. spiralis*, which recognize their residues of tivelosa [51, 59, 62]. These TSL-1 antigens induce the maturation and activation of dendritic cells, which leads to the presentation of antigen, through the expression of the major histocompatibility complex (MHC) class II [63, 64], promoting the development of the Th1 type immune response [48], with the subsequent predominance of a Th2 type immune response, resulting in a mixture of both Th1/Th2 immune responses, dependent on the CD4$^+$ T cells (**Figure 4**) [65, 66].

The Th1 type immune response against *T. spiralis* is characterized by a significant increase in Th1 cytokines such as IL-12 [67–69], INF-γ [48, 67–70], IL-1β [69, 71] and TNF-α (**Figure 4**) [67–69, 72]. In recent years, studies have shown that the production of Th1 cytokines is directly associated with the development of the inflammatory response and intestinal pathology, which favors the infection by *T. spiralis*. IL-12 and INF-γ participate in the polarization of the Th1 immune response [48, 67, 68]. IL-12 promotes the differentiation of *naive* T cells to a Th1 phenotype that produces INF-γ [73], which induces the expression of MHC II molecules in dendritic cells [74], increases the development and differentiation of Th1 cells, induces the expression of transcription factors such as nuclear factor (NF)-κB [75] and regulates the production of proinflammatory cytokines [76, 77]. However, exogenous administration of IL-12 in *T. spiralis* infection suppresses intestinal mastocytosis, delaying the expulsion of the parasite and increasing the parasitic muscle burden [78]. TNF-α is a potent proinflammatory cytokine [79], which plays a key role in the pathogenesis of inflammatory diseases, since it participates in the activation of a cascade of proinflammatory cytokines, such as IL-1β [79–81]. Studies have shown that the production of TNF-α during infection by *T. spiralis* is associated with the development of intestinal pathology [72, 82–84]. TNF-α also induces the expression of iNOS and consequently NO production [85–88], which acts mainly as an effector molecule in against both extracellular and intracellular parasites [89]. Studies have shown that TSL-1 antigens are capable to induce the expression of iNOS with the consequent production of NO [90]. However, NO production is also associated with the development of intestinal pathology in *T. spiralis* infection [72, 91]. Finally, IL-1β is a proinflammatory cytokine [92, 93], which is produced during infection by *T. spiralis*, participating in the inflammatory bowel response. However, until now, its function is not well known [69, 71].

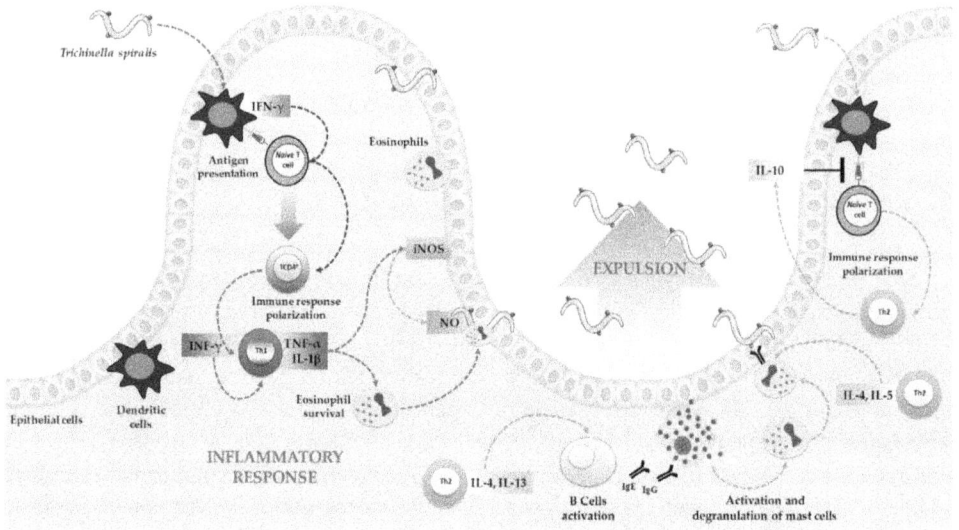

Figure 4. Immune response against *Trichinella spiralis*. TSL-1 antigens of *T. spiralis* induced the dendritic cells maturation, polarizing initially a Th1 immune response, which is mainly characterized by the release of IL-12, INF-γ, NO, IL-1β and TNF-α, and developing inflammatory intestinal response, which results in the development of intestinal pathology. Moreover, the TSL-1 antigens of *T. spiralis* can also induce a Th2 immune response, characterized by the release of IL-4, IL-5, IL-10 and IL-13, eosinophil and mast cells hyperplasia, favoring *T. spiralis* expulsion.

On the other hand, TSL-1 antigens are capable of activating dendritic cells and CD4$^+$ T cells [63, 94], inducing the synthesis of Th2 cytokines such as IL-4, IL-5, IL-10 and IL-13 (**Figure 4**) [48, 67, 68, 70, 95–97]. IL-4 and IL-5 [98] are a critical factor in the terminal differentiation and proliferation of eosinophils, which are involved in the development of intestinal pathology, thus promoting the inflammatory response during infection by *T. spiralis* [14, 99]. IL-4 plays a central role in regulating the differentiation of antigen-stimulated *naïve* T cells, causing such cells to develop into Th2 cells capable of producing IL-4 and several other Th2 cytokines including IL-5, IL-10 and IL-13. In addition, it suppresses potently the production of INF-γ [100, 101]. IL-10 is a cytokine of great importance during infection by *T. spiralis*, which decreases the production of IL-12, IFN-γ and the proliferation and presentation of antigens of dendritic cells, polarizing the immune response to Th2 type [65, 102]. Since the absence or decrease of IL-10 significantly delays the intestinal expulsion of *T. spiralis*, increasing the muscular parasite burden [78]. IL-13 is also a cytokine produced by Th2 cells, which has direct effects on eosinophils, including the promotion of their survival, activation and recruitment [103–105]. The synthesis and release of IL-4 and IL-13 induce B cell proliferation and the expression of surface antigens, including the CD23 receptor (FcεRII) of low affinity to IgE and MHC class II molecules, stimulating the production of IgE [106, 107]; inducing hyperplasia of mast cells and eosinophils, which triggers immediate hypersensitivity reactions [108–110]; rapidly expanding in the mucosa, predominantly within the epithelium [63], where the TSL-1 antigens can directly induce their degranulation; and promoting the expulsion of *T. spiralis* from the intestine [51]. Studies in mice deficient in IL-4/IL-13 showed a reduction in the expulsion of *T. spiralis* and mastocytosis, showing development of intestinal pathology [82, 83, 111].

6. Diagnosis of Trichinellosis

The early clinical diagnosis of Trichinellosis is quite difficult due to the lack of symptoms and pathognomonic signs. In addition, chronic forms of the disease are not easy to diagnose [14]. When the infection occurs in epizootic or outbreak form, its diagnosis is easier. However, it is difficult in low-level or sporadic infections, since the clinical picture is usually common to many other enteric diseases. This makes it necessary to carry out a differential diagnosis [34]. The diagnosis of Trichinellosis must be based on three main criteria: (1) clinical findings—recognition of signs and symptoms; (2) laboratory parameters, such as eosinophilia and muscle enzymes, detection of antibodies and/or detection of L1-*T. spiralis* in muscle biopsy and (3) epidemiological research—idemtification of the source and origin of the infection and outbreak studies [14].

Identification of L1-*T. spiralis* in muscle tissue is the positive diagnosis of the disease; any technique used for this purpose is included within the so-called Direct Diagnostic Methods [42], which performed post-mortem and includes four main techniques: (1) plate compression [72], (2) polymerase chain reaction (PCR) [14, 36], (3) artificial or enzymatic digestion [72] and (4) histology [24]. The detection of antibodies against *T. spiralis* in the host represents a solid evidence of contact with the parasite, and the techniques developed for that purpose are included among the Indirect Diagnostic Methods [42], through which they are detected antibodies against *T. spiralis* antigens. Among which we find (1) indirect immunofluorescence [112], (2) enzyme-linked immunosorbent assay (ELISA), (3) Western blot [113] and 4) microimmunodiffusion double [40].

7. Treatment of Trichinellosis

7.1. Pharmacotherapy

Pharmacotherapy used in Trichinellosis includes the use of antiparasitic and steroidal anti-inflammatory drugs [114]. Currently, the antiparasitic treatment used for Trichinellosis is the administration of benzimidazoles, mainly albendazole and mebendazole, which are effective against the parasite [40, 115]. In addition, different antiparasitic drugs such as ivermectin, nitazoxanide, quinfamide and flubendazole have been evaluated, and favorable results have been observed [40, 116]. These drugs are the most effective therapies at the beginning of the disease, since they kill the adult parasites. Although albendazole is better tolerated, a recent research showed that thiabendazole was a potent and curable drug because its efficacy was almost 100% to eliminate intestinal worms [117].

Respect to pharmacotherapy with steroidal anti-inflammatory drugs, glucocorticoids (GC) are the most used for the treatment of signs and symptoms of the inflammatory response produced by the *T. spiralis* infection [118, 119]. GC are potent anti-inflammatory drugs, which regulate transcriptional pathways in diverse cellular contexts such as development, homeostasis, metabolism and inflammation [120]. GC exert their anti-inflammatory activity primarily in two ways: (1) induce the expression of several genes that encode proteins that exert anti-inflammatory effects such as the leukocyte-inhibitory secretory protein, the inhibitor of NF-κB (IκB-α), IL-10 and the IL-1 antagonist receptor [121, 122]; (2) inhibit the expression of proinflammatory genes by suppression of transcription factors, such as NF-κB [123] and activating protein (AP)-1 [120], through the protein-protein interaction [124], regulating the inflammatory cytokines expression, such as TNF-α, IL-1α, IL-1β, IL-8, IFN-α and IFN-β, and inflammatory enzymes such as iNOS, cyclooxygenase (COX)-2, inducible phospholipase A2 (cPLA2), adhesion molecules and inflammatory receptors [125, 126].

Although GCs are potent anti-inflammatory drugs, their therapeutic use in Trichinellosis is limited [127], since research in recent years has shown that treatment with betamethasone [128] and dexamethasone [129] increases the parasitic load at the muscular level. Recently, studies showed that treatment with dexamethasone in the intestinal phase of *T. spiralis* infection inhibited the production of inflammatory mediators, such as PGE_2, NO, TNF-α, IL-1β, IL-12 and INF-γ, decreasing the number of eosinophils in the blood and the development of intestinal pathology. However, in the muscular phase, the implantation and parasite burden of L1-*T. spiralis* increased significantly [69, 72].

Given this therapeutic problem, new pharmacological strategies have been developed in the use of new anti-inflammatory drugs, which help to inhibit the inflammatory response during Trichinellosis, without the GC side effects. Resiniferatoxin is a vanilloid derived from the cactus plant *Euphoria resiniferous*, an agonist of the transient receptor potential vanilloid (TRPV)-1 [130], which activates and then desensitizes the TRPV1 receptor producing an analgesic effect [131, 132]. Studies in both models *in vitro* and *in vivo* have shown that resiniferatoxin has an important anti-inflammatory activity, inhibiting the expression of NF-κB [133], iNOS and COX-2 [134], and the synthesis of PGE_2, NO and TNF-α [135, 136]. Finally, recent studies showed that treatment with resiniferatoxin during the intestinal phase of infection by *T. spiralis* decreased the levels of PGE_2, NO, TNF-α, Il-1β, IL-12 and INF-γ, as well as the number of eosinophils in blood. While in the muscular phase of *T. spiralis* infection, treatment with resiniferatoxin significantly decreased implantation and parasite burden of L1-*T. spiralis* [69, 72]. These findings suggest that resiniferatoxin may be a potential drug in the treatment of inflammatory diseases.

7.2. Immunotherapy

In immunotherapy during Trichinellosis, total and immunodominant antigens have been used, which activate the immune system of the host, causing a decrease in parasite burden in the intestine, affecting the fecundity of adult female worms, thus impacting the parasite burden on muscle tissue [137, 138]. Studies have shown that immunotherapy with *T. spiralis* total soluble (TS) antigen in murine experimental models induces protection, since a decrease in muscle parasite burden was observed [139]. In a study based on pig model infected with *T. spiralis*, to which immunotherapy was applied with *T. spiralis* TS antigen, antigens were identified in a molecular weight range of 14–97 kDa. Immunotherapy with *T. spiralis* TS antigen provoked a primary immune response, with a reduction in parasite burden, as well as damage to CN in the muscular phase of the infection, compared with the control group (without immunotherapy) [140].

On the other hand, TS and 45 kDa antigens of *T. spiralis* have been used [141], obtaining a greater protective effect on the part of the 45 kDa antigen, since it was observed alteration of the NC. Thus, 45-kDa immunodominant antigen has been shown to be the most effective antigen against *T. spiralis* infection [142]. However, research with this immunodominant antigen continues to be viable as a vaccine in the future.

Immunization with 45 kDa antigens of *T. spiralis* has produced important effects on the immune response in the murine model, such is the case of immunization applied in rats with different nutritional conditions, which showed decreased parasite burden compared to controls becoming null in the nourished rats. In this study, *T. spiralis* TS antigen was applied in nourished and malnourished rats, which decreased the parasite burden in comparison with controls without treatment, observing lower parasite burden in nourished rats. *T. spiralis* TS antigen provoked an immune response against the *L1-T. spiralis*, since not only decreases the parasite burden but also causes changes at the histological level of the NC and prevented the implant, as occurred in the immunization with the 45-kDa antigen in nourished rats, conferring a high level of protection [141]. Similarly, in another study applying immunotherapy with TS and 45 kDa antigens of *T. spiralis*, a reduction in parasite burden was observed [16, 112].

A study in a rat model, in which the sublingual immunization treatment was applied with *T. spiralis* TS antigen, vehicle for sublingual immunotherapy (VSIT) and polyvalent bacterial vaccine, a protection against the infection of *T. spiralis* was observed [143]. Currently, adjuvants are substances that stimulate or improve the immune response against an antigen, without having a specific antigenic effect by themselves. The function of the adjuvant is determinant to achieve an adequate immune response. Encouraging results have been obtained in immunotherapy with the 45 kDa antigen adding an adjuvant. For what is believed to be a good therapeutic alternative through the sublingual route for the treatment of Trichinellosis.

8. Conclusion

Currently, Trichinellosis is a reemerging zoonotic parasitic disease that continues to affect the health of both animals and humans worldwide. For this reason, it is important to know well the biology of its etiological agent *Trichinella*, as well as its mechanisms of evasion of the host's immune system, with the purpose of making a timely and differential diagnosis, to achieve a good treatment. Simultaneously, it is necessary to continue investigating therapeutic strategies that, through pharmacotherapy and immunotherapy, develop specific treatments directed to the parasite, avoiding collateral effects to the host.

Acknowledgements

Thanks to the authors who collaborated in the writing of this chapter: Dr. José Luis Muñoz, Claudia Maldonado, Argelia López, José Jesús Muñoz, Juan Armando Flores and Alejandra Moreno, as well as the Universities involved: Cuauhtémoc University Aguascalientes and Autonomous University of Zacatecas. Thanks for the financial support for chapter publication.

Conflict of interest

We have no conflict of interest related to this work.

Author details

José Luis Muñoz-Carrillo[1]*, Claudia Maldonado-Tapia[2], Argelia López-Luna[3],
José Jesús Muñoz-Escobedo[4], Juan Armando Flores-De La Torre[3] and
Alejandra Moreno-García[2]

*Address all correspondence to: mcbjlmc@gmail.com

1 Faculty of Odontology, School of Biomedical Sciences of the Cuauhtémoc University
Aguascalientes, Aguascalientes, Mexico

2 Laboratory of Cell Biology and Microbiology, Academic Unit of Biological Sciences,
Autonomous University of Zacatecas, Zacatecas, Mexico

3 Laboratory of Pharmacy and Toxicology, Autonomous University of Zacatecas, Zacatecas,
Mexico

4 Academic Unit of Odontology, Autonomous University of Zacatecas, Zacatecas, Mexico

References

[1] Babu S, Nutman TB. Immune responses to helminth infection. In: Rich RR, Fleisher TA, Shearer WT, Schroeder HW, Frew AJ, Weyand CM, editors. Clinical Immunology. 5th ed. London: Elsevier; 2019. pp. 437-447.e1. DOI: 10.1016/B978-0-7020-6896-6.00031-4

[2] Grencis RK, Humphreys NE, Bancroft AJ. Immunity to gastrointestinal nematodes: Mechanisms and myths. Immunological Reviews. 2014;**260**(1):183-205. DOI: 10.1111/imr.12188

[3] McSorley HJ, Maizels RM. Helminth infections and host immune regulation. Clinical Microbiology Reviews. 2012;**25**(4):585-608. DOI: 10.1128/CMR.05040-11

[4] Maizels RM, Hewitson JP, Smith KA. Susceptibility and immunity to helminth parasites. Current Opinion in Immunology. 2012;**24**(4):459-466. DOI: 10.1016/j.coi.2012.06.003

[5] Zaph C, Cooper PJ, Harris NL. Mucosal immune responses following intestinal nematode infection. Parasite Immunology. 2014;**36**(9):439-452. DOI: 10.1111/pim.12090

[6] Maizels RM, Yazdanbakhsh M. Immune regulation by helminth parasites: Cellular and molecular mechanisms. Nature Reviews. Immunology. 2003;**3**(9):733-744. DOI: 10.1038/nri1183

[7] Elliott DE, Summers RW, Weinstock JV. Helminths as governors of immune-mediated inflammation. International Journal for Parasitology. 2007;**37**(5):457-464. DOI: 10.1016/j. ijpara.2006.12.009

[8] Bruschi F, Chiumiento L. Immunomodulation in trichinellosis: Does *Trichinella* really escape the host immune system? Endocrine, Metabolic & Immune Disorders Drug Targets. 2012;**12**(1):4-15. DOI: 10.2174/187153012799279081

[9] Pozio E. World distribution of *Trichinella spp*. infections in animals and humans. Veterinary Parasitology. 2007;**149**(1–2):3-21. DOI: 10.1016/j.vetpar.2007.07.002

[10] Muñoz-Carrillo JL, Contreras-Cordero JF, Muñoz-López JL, Maldonado-Tapia CH, Muñoz-Escobedo JJ, Moreno-García MA. Cover image. Parasite Immunology. 2017;**39**(9). DOI: 10.1111/pim.12457

[11] Krivokapich SJ, Pozio E, Gatti GM, Prous CL, Ribicich M, Marucci G, et al. *Trichinella patagoniensis* n. sp. (Nematoda), a new encapsulated species infecting carnivorous mammals in South America. International Journal for Parasitology. 2012;**42**(10):903-910. DOI: 10.1016/j.ijpara.2012.07.009

[12] Pozio E, Zarlenga DS. New pieces of the *Trichinella* puzzle. International Journal for Parasitology. 2013;**43**(12–13):983-997. DOI: 10.1016/j.ijpara.2013.05.010

[13] Korhonen PK, Pozio E, La Rosa G, Chang BC, Koehler AV, Hoberg EP, et al. Phylogenomic and biogeographic reconstruction of the Trichinella complex. Nature Communications. 2016;**7**:10513. DOI: 10.1038/ncomms10513

[14] Gottstein B, Pozio E, Nöckler K. 2009. Epidemiology, diagnosis, treatment, and control of trichinellosis. Clinical Microbiology Reviews. 2009;**22**(1):127-145. DOI: 10.1128/CMR.000 26-08

[15] Bruschi F. Trichinellosis in developing countries: Is it neglected? Journal of Infection in Developing Countries. 2012;**6**(3):216-222. DOI: 10.3855/jidc.2478

[16] Alejandra MGM. Epidemiología, diagnóstico y tratamiento de la Trichinellosis en México. España:. Editorial Académica Española; 2018. p. 4. ISBN: 3841754503, 9783841754509

[17] Builes Cuartas LM, Laverde Trujillo LM. Triquinelosis una zoonosis parasitaria (trichinellosis a parasitic zoonosis). CES Medicina Veterinaria & Zootecnica. 2009;**4**(2):130-136

[18] Berger SA. Trichinosis: Global Status: 2017 Edition. GIDEON Informatics Inc.; 2017. pp. 1-114. e-books. ISBN: 978-1-4988-1680-9

[19] Pozio E. 2014. Searching for *Trichinella*: Not all pigs are created equal. Trends in Parasitology. 2014;**30**(1):4-11. DOI: 10.1016/j.pt.2013.11.001

[20] Cervera-Castillo H, Torres-Caballero V, Martínez-García E, Blanco-Favela FA. Triquinosis humana. Un caso que simula polimiositis. Revista Médica del Instituto Mexicano del Seguro Social. 2009;**47**(3):323-326

[21] FAO/WHO. Identifican los diez principales parásitos transmitidos por los alimentos [Internet]. 2014. Available from: http://www.fao.org/news/story/es/item/237578/icode/ [Accessed: Jun 7, 2018]

[22] Calcagno MA, Teixeira C, Forastiero MA, Costantino SN, Venturiello SM. Aspectos clínicos, serológicos y parasitológicos de un brote de Trichinellosis humana en Villa Mercedes, San Luis, Argentina. Medicina (Buenos Aires). 2005;**65**(4):302-306. ISSN: 1669-9106

[23] Berger SA. Infectious Diseases of Mexico, 2010. GIDEON Informatics Inc.; 2010. e-books. p. 439

[24] Chávez MI, Reveles RG, Muñoz JJ, Maldonado C, Moreno MA. Utilidad del modelo experimental de cerdo en el estudio y tratamiento de la Trichinellosis. REDVET: Revista Electrónica de Veterinaria. 2011;**12**(5B):1-18. ISSN: 1695-7504

[25] SINAVE: Sistema Nacional de Vigilancia Epidemiológica. Boletín Epidemiológico [Internet]. 2016;**47**(33):1-68. Available from: https://www.gob.mx/cms/uploads/attachment/file/170938/sem47.pdf [Accessed: Jun 7, 2018]

[26] Berger SA. Infectious Diseases of Mexico: 2017 Edition. GIDEON Informatics Inc.; 2017. p. 368-369. e-books. ISBN: 978-1-4988-1412-6

[27] Ortega-Pierres MG. Triquinelosis. Revista Ciencia-Academia Mexicana de Ciencias. 2017;**68**(1):74-77

[28] Berumen de la Torre V, Muñoz Escobedo JJ, Moreno García MA. Trichinellosis en perros callejeros de la ciudad de Zacatecas, México. Parasitología latinoamericana. 2002;**57**(1–2): 72-74. ISSN: 0717-7712

[29] Moreno GA, Rivas GJ, Berumen TV, Muñoz EJ. Detección de *Trichinella spiralis* en rata domestica del basurero municipal de Zacatecas. REDVET: Revista Electrónica de Veterinaria. 2007;**8**(5):1-8. ISSN: 1695-7504

[30] Tapia M, Bracamontes Maldonado N, López Bernal S, Muñoz Escobedo J, Chávez Guajardo E, Moreno García A. Anti-*T. spiralis* Antibodies Detection in some Localities of Zacatecas (México). International Archives of Medicine. 2015;**8**(216):1-6. DOI: 10.3823/1815

[31] Owen R. Description of a microscophc entozoon infesting the muscles of the human body. Journal of Zoology. 1835;**1**(4):315-324. DOI: 10.1111/j.1096-3642.1835.tb00631.x

[32] Cox FEG. History of human parasitology. Clinical Microbiology Reviews. 2002;**15**(4):595-612. DOI: 10.1128/CMR.15.4.595-612.2002

[33] Pozio E. Factors affecting the flow among domestic, synanthropic and sylvatic cycles of *Trichinella*. Veterinary Parasitology. 2000;**93**(3–4):241-262. DOI: 10.1016/S0304-4017(00)00344-7

[34] Bruschi F, Murrell KD. New aspects of human trichinellosis: The impact of new *Trichinella* species. Postgraduate Medical Journal. 2002;**78**(915):15-22. DOI: 10.1136/pmj.78.915.15

[35] Murrell KD. The dynamics of *Trichinella spiralis* epidemiology: Out to pasture? Veterinary Parasitology. 2016;**231**:92-96. DOI: 10.1016/j.vetpar.2016.03.020

[36] Despommier DD, Gwadz RW, Hotez PJ, Charles AK. Parasitic Diseases. 5th ed. Apple Trees Productions; 2005. pp. 135-142

[37] Theodoropoulos G, Petrakos G. *Trichinella spiralis*: Differential effect of host bile on the in vitro invasion of infective larvae into epithelial cells. Experimental Parasitology. 2010; **126**(4):441-444. DOI: 10.1016/j.exppara.2010.05.013

[38] Mitreva M, Jasmer DP. Biology and genome of *Trichinella spiralis*. WormBook. 2006:1-21. DOI: 10.1895/wormbook.1.124.1

[39] Moreno García MA, Maldonado Tapia CH, García Mayorga EA, Reveles Hernández RG, Muñoz Escobedo JJ. Fase Intestinal de *Trichinella spiralis* en modelo murino. Acta Biológica Colombiana. 2009;**14**(1):203-210. ISSN: 0120-548X

[40] Moreno AG, Maldonado CT, Chávez Ruvalcaba IR, Reveles RGH, Núñez QZ, Muñoz JJE. El estudio de *Trichinella spiralis* en modelos experimentales. REDVET: Revista Electrónica de Veterinaria. 2012;**13**(7):1-12. ISSN: 1695-7504

[41] Wu Z, Sofronic-Milosavljevic LJ, Nagano I, Takahashi Y. *Trichinella spiralis*: Nurse cell formation with emphasis on analogy to muscle cell repair. Parasites & Vectors. 2008;**1**(1): 1-27. DOI: 10.1186/1756-3305-1-27

[42] Laverde LM, Builes LM, Masso CJ. Detección de *Trichinella spiralis* en cerdos faenados en dos plantas de beneficio en el municipio de bello. Revista CES. Medicina Veterinaria y Zootecnia. 2009;**4**(2):47-56. ISSN: 1900-9607

[43] Pozio E, Paterlini F, Pedarra C, Sacchi L, Bugarini R, Goffredo E, et al. Predilection sites of *Trichinella spiralis* larvae in naturally infected horses. Journal of Helminthology. 1999; **73**(3):233-237. PMID: 10526416

[44] Kapel CM, Webster P, Gamble HR. Muscle distribution of sylvatic and domestic *Trichinella* larvae in production animals and wildlife. Veterinary Parasitology. 2005;**132** (1–2):101-105. DOI: 10.1016/j.vetpar.2005.05.036

[45] Ribicich M, Rosa A, Bolpe J, Scialfa E, Cardillo N, Pasqualetti MI, et al. Avances en el estudio del diagnóstico y la prevención de la Trichinellosis. Jornadas de la Asociación Argentina de Parasitología Veterinaria y XIX Encuentro Rioplatense de Veterinarios Endoparasitólogos. 2010:1-6

[46] Chávez Guajardo EG, Saldivar Elías S, Muñoz Escobedo JJ, Moreno García MA. Trichinellosis una zoonosis vigente. REDVET: Revista Electrónica de Veterinaria. 2006; 7(6):1-19. ISSN: 1695-7504

[47] Murrell KD, Pozio E. Worldwide occurrence and impact of human trichinellosis, 1986-2009. Emerging Infectious Diseases. 2011;**17**(12):2194-2202. DOI: 10.3201/eid1712.110896

[48] Gruden-Movsesijan A, Ilic N, Colic M, Majstorovic I, Vasilev S, Radovic I, et al. The impact of *Trichinella spiralis* excretory-secretory products on dendritic cells. Comparative Immunology, Microbiology and Infectious Diseases. 2011;**34**(5):429-439. DOI: 10.1016/j.cimid.2011.08.004

[49] Ortega-Pierres MG, Yepez-Mulia L, Homan W, Gamble HR, Lim PL, Takahashi Y, et al. Workshop on a detailed characterization of *Trichinella spiralis* antigens: A platform for future studies on antigens and antibodies to this parasite. Parasite Immunology. 1996;**18**(6):273-284. DOI: 10.1046/j.1365-3024.1996.d01-103.x

[50] Appleton JA, Romaris F. A pivotal role for glycans at the interface between *Trichinella spiralis* and its host. Veterinary Parasitology. 2001;**101**(3–4):249-260. DOI: 10.1016/S0304-4017(01)00570-2

[51] Yépez-Mulia L, Hernández-Bello R, Arizmendi-Puga N, Ortega-Pierres G. Contributions to the study of *Trichinella spiralis* TSL-1 antigens in host immunity. Parasite Immunology. 2007;**29**(12):661-670

[52] Gold AM, Despommier DD, Buck SW. Partial characterization of two antigens secreted by L1 larvae of *Trichinella spiralis*. Molecular and Biochemical Parasitology. 1990;**41**(2):187-196. DOI: 10.1016/0166-6851(90)90181-K

[53] Su XZ, Prestwood AK, McGraw RA. Cloning and expression of complementary DNA encoding an antigen of *Trichinella spiralis*. Molecular and Biochemical Parasitology. 1991;**45**(2):331-336. DOI: 10.1016/0166-6851(91)90101-B

[54] Wu Z, Nagano I, Nakada T, Takahashi Y. Expression of excretory and secretory protein genes of *Trichinella* at muscle stage differs before and after cyst formation. Parasitology International. 2002;**51**(2):155-161. DOI: 10.1016/S1383-5769(02)00003-X

[55] Mitreva M, Jasmer DP, Appleton J, Martin J, Dante M, Wylie T, et al. Gene discovery in the adenophorean nematode *Trichinella spiralis*: An analysis of transcription from three life cycle stages. Molecular and Biochemical Parasitology. 2004;**137**(2):277-291. DOI: 10.1016/j.molbiopara.2004.05.015

[56] Zarlenga DS, Gamble HR. Molecular cloning and expression of an immunodominant 53-kDa excretory-secretory antigen from *Trichinella spiralis* muscle larvae. Molecular and Biochemical Parasitology. 1990;**42**(2):165-174. DOI: 10.1016/0166-6851(90)90159-J

[57] Zarlenga DS, Gamble HR. Molecular cloning and expression of an immunodominant 53-kDa excretory-secretory antigen from *Trichinella spiralis* muscle larvae. Molecular and Biochemical Parasitology. 1995;**72**(1–2):253. DOI: 10.1016/0166-6851(95)00071-8

[58] Romarís F, Escalante M, Lorenzo S, Bonay P, Gárate T, Leiro J, et al. Monoclonal antibodies raised in Btk(xid) mice reveal new antigenic relationships and molecular interactions among gp53 and other *Trichinella* glycoproteins. Molecular and Biochemical Parasitology. 2002;**125**(1–2):173-183. DOI: 10.1016/S0166-6851(02)00239-6

[59] Nagano I, Wu Z, Takahashi Y. Functional genes and proteins of *Trichinella* spp. Parasitology Research. 2009;**104**(2):197-207. DOI: 10.1007/s00436-008-1248-1

[60] Arasu P, Ellis LA, Iglesias R, Ubeira FM, Appleton JA. Molecular analysis of antigens targeted by protective antibodies in rapid expulsion of *Trichinella spiralis*. Molecular and Biochemical Parasitology. 1994;**65**(2):201-211. DOI: 10.1016/0166-6851(94)90072-8

[61] Beiting DP, Gagliardo LF, Hesse M, Bliss SK, Meskill D, Appleton JA. Coordinated control of immunity to muscle stage *Trichinella spiralis* by IL-10, regulatory T cells, and TGF-beta. Journal of Immunology. 2007;**178**(2):1039-1047. DOI: 10.4049/jimmunol.178.2.1039

[62] Reason AJ, Ellis LA, Appleton JA, Wisnewski N, Grieve RB, McNeil M, et al. 1994. Novel tyvelose-containing tri- and tetra-antennary N-glycans in the immunodominant antigens of the intracellular parasite *Trichinella spiralis*. Glycobiology. 1994;**4**(5):593-603. DOI: 10.1093/glycob/4.5.593

[63] Ilic N, Worthington JJ, Gruden-Movsesijan A, Travis MA, Sofronic-Milosavljevic L, Grencis RK. *Trichinella spiralis* antigens prime mixed Th1/Th2 response but do not induce de novo generation of Foxp3+ T cells in vitro. Parasite Immunology. 2011;**33**(10):572-582. DOI: 10.1111/j.1365-3024.2011.01322.x

[64] Sofronic-Milosavljevic L, Ilic N, Pinelli E, Gruden-Movsesijan A. Secretory products of *Trichinella spiralis* muscle larvae and immunomodulation: Implication for autoimmune diseases, allergies, and malignancies. Journal of Immunology Research. 2015;**2015**:523 875. DOI: 10.1155/2015/523875

[65] Ilic N, Gruden-Movsesijan A, Sofronic-Milosavljevic L. *Trichinella spiralis*: Shaping the immune response. Immunologic Research. 2012;**52**(1–2):111-119. DOI: 10.1007/s12026-012-8287-5

[66] Ashour DS. *Trichinella spiralis* immunomodulation: An interactive multifactorial process. Expert Review of Clinical Immunology. 2013;**9**(7):669-675. DOI: 10.1586/1744666X.2013. 811187

[67] Gentilini MV, Nuñez GG, Roux ME, Venturiello SM. Trichinella spiralis infection rapidly induces lung inflammatory response: The lung as the site of helminthocytotoxic activity. Immunobiology. 2011;**216**(9):1054-1063. DOI: 10.1016/j.imbio.2011.02.002

[68] Yu YR, Deng MJ, Lu WW, Jia MZ, Wu W, Qi YF. Systemic cytokine profiles and splenic toll-like receptor expression during Trichinella spiralis infection. Experimental Parasitology. 2013;**134**(1):92-101. DOI: 10.1016/j.exppara.2013.02.014

[69] Muñoz-Carrillo JL, Contreras-Cordero JF, Muñoz-López JL, Maldonado-Tapia CH, Muñoz-Escobedo JJ, Moreno-García MA. Resiniferatoxin modulates the Th1 immune response and protects the host during intestinal nematode infection. Parasite Immunology. 2017;**39**(9):1-16. DOI: 10.1111/pim.12448

[70] Ilic N, Colic M, Gruden-Movsesijan A, Majstorovic I, Vasilev S, Sofronic-Milosavljevic LJ. Characterization of rat bone marrow dendritic cells initially primed by *Trichinella spiralis* antigens. Parasite Immunology. 2008;**30**(9):491-495. DOI: 10.1111/j.1365-3024.2008.01049.x

[71] Ming L, Peng RY, Zhang L, Zhang CL, Lv P, Wang ZQ, et al. Invasion by Trichinella spiralis infective larvae affects the levels of inflammatory cytokines in intestinal epithelial cells in vitro. Experimental Parasitology. 2016;**170**:220-226. DOI: 10.1016/j.exppara.2016.10.003

[72] Muñoz-Carrillo JL, Muñoz-Escobedo JJ, Maldonado-Tapia CH, Chávez-Ruvalcaba F, Moreno-García MA. Resiniferatoxin lowers TNF-α, NO and PGE$_2$ in the intestinal phase and the parasite burden in the muscular phase of *Trichinella spiralis* infection. Parasite Immunology. 2017;**39**(1):1-14. DOI: 10.1111/pim.12393

[73] Teng MW, Bowman EP, McElwee JJ, Smyth MJ, Casanova JL, Cooper AM, et al. IL-12 and IL-23 cytokines: From discovery to targeted therapies for immune-mediated inflammatory diseases. Nature Medicine. 2015;**21**(7):719-729. DOI: 10.1038/nm.389

[74] Pestka S, Krause CD, Walter MR. Interferons, interferon-like cytokines, and their receptors. Immunological Reviews. 2004;**202**:8-32. DOI: 10.1111/j.0105-2896.2004.00204.x

[75] Mühl H, Pfeilschifter J. Anti-inflammatory properties of pro-inflammatory interferon-γ. International Immunopharmacology. 2003;**3**(9):1247-1255. DOI: 10.1016/S1567-5769(03) 00131-0

[76] Neumann B, Emmanuilidis K, Stadler M, Holzmann B. Distinct functions of interferon-gamma for chemokine expression in models of acute lung inflammation. Immunology. 1998;**95**(4):512-521. DOI: 10.1046/j.1365-2567.1998.00643.x

[77] Muñoz-Carrillo JL, Ortega-Martín Del Campo J, Gutiérrez-Coronado O, Villalobos-Gutiérrez PT, Contreras-Cordero JF, Ventura-Juárez J. Adipose tissue and inflammation. In: Szablewski L, editor. Adipose Tissue. InTech; 2018. pp. 93-121. DOI: 10.5772/intechopen. 74227

[78] Helmby H, Grencis RK. IFN-γ-independent effects of IL-12 during intestinal nematode infection. Journal of Immunology. 2003;**171**(7):3691-3696. DOI: 10.4049/jimmunol.171. 7.3691

[79] Leung L. Cahill CM, TNF-α and neuropathic pain-a review. Journal of Neuroinflammation. 2010;**7**:27. DOI: 10.1186/1742-2094-7-27

[80] Horiuchi T, Mitoma H, Harashima SI, Tsukamoto H, Shimoda T. Transmembrane TNF-α: Structure, function and interaction with anti-TNF agents. Rheumatology (Oxford, England). 2010;**49**(7):1215-1228. DOI: 10.1093/rheumatology/keq031

[81] Parameswaran N, Patial S. Tumor necrosis factor-α signaling in macrophages. Critical Reviews in Eukaryotic Gene Expression. 2010;**20**:87-103. PMID: 21133840

[82] Lawrence CE, Paterson JC, Higgins LM, MacDonald TT, Kennedy MW, Garside P. IL-4-regulated enteropathy in an intestinal nematode infection. European Journal of Immunology. 1998;**28**(9):2672-2684. DOI: 10.1002/(SICI)1521-4141(199809)28:09<2672::AID-IMMU2672>3.0.CO;2-F

[83] Ierna MX, Scales HE, Saunders KL, Lawrence CE. Mast cell production of IL-4 and TNF may be required for protective and pathological responses in gastrointestinal helminth infection. Mucosal Immunology. 2008;**1**(2):147-155. DOI: 10.1038/mi.2007.16

[84] Ierna MX, Scales HE, Müller C, Lawrence CE. Transmembrane tumor necrosis factor alpha is required for enteropathy and is sufficient to promote parasite expulsion in

gastrointestinal helminth infection. Infection and Immunity. 2009;**77**(9):3879-3885. DOI: 10.1128/IAI.01461-08

[85] Bogdan C. Nitric oxide and the immune response. Nature Immunology. 2001;**2**(10):907-916. DOI: 10.1038/ni1001-907

[86] Guzik TJ, Korbut R, Adamek-Guzik T. Nitric oxide and superoxide in inflammation and immune regulation. Journal of Physiology and Pharmacology. 2003;**54**(4):469-487. PMID: 14726604

[87] Marzocco S, Di Paola R, Serraino I, Sorrentino R, Meli R, Mattaceraso G, et al. Effect of methylguanidine in carrageenan-induced acute inflammation in the rats. European Journal of Pharmacology. 2004;**484**:341-350

[88] Wink DA, Hines HB, Cheng RYS, Switzer CH, Flores-Santana W, Vitek MP, et al. Nitric oxide and redox mechanisms in the immune response. Journal of Leukocyte Biology. 2011;**89**(6):873-891. DOI: 10.1189/jlb.1010550

[89] Moncada S, Erusalimsky JD. Does nitric oxide modulate mitochondrial energy generation and apoptosis? Nature Reviews. Molecular Cell Biology. 2002;**3**(3):214-220. DOI: 10.1038/nrm762

[90] Andrade MA, Siles-Lucas M, López-Abán J, Nogal-Ruiz JJ, Pérez-Arellano JL, Martínez-Fernández AR, et al. *Trichinella*: Differing effects of antigens from encapsulated and non-encapsulated species on in vitro nitric oxide production. Veterinary Parasitology. 2007;**143**(1):86-90. DOI: 10.1016/j.vetpar.2006.07.026

[91] Lawrence CE, Paterson JC, Wei XQ, Liew FY, Garside P, Kennedy MW. Nitric oxide mediates intestinal pathology but not immune expulsion during *Trichinella spiralis* infection in mice. Journal of Immunology. 2000;**164**(8):4229-4234. DOI: 10.4049/jimmunol.164.8.4229

[92] Dinarello CA. Immunological and inflammatory functions of the interleukin-1 family. Annual Review of Immunology. 2009;**27**:519-550. DOI: 10.1146/annurev.immunol.021908.132612

[93] Garib FY, Rizopulu AP, Kuchmiy AA, Garib VF. Inactivation of inflammasomes by pathogens regulates inflammation. Biochemistry (Mosc). 2016;**81**(11):1326-1339. DOI: 10.1134/S0006297916110109

[94] Sofronic-Milosavljevic LJ, Radovic I, Ilic N, Majstorovic I, Cvetkovic J, Gruden-Movsesijan A. Application of dendritic cells stimulated with *Trichinella spiralis* excretory-secretory antigens alleviates experimental autoimmune encephalomyelitis. Medical Microbiology and Immunology. 2013;**202**(3):239-249. DOI: 10.1007/s00430-012-0286-6

[95] Roy A, Sawesi O, Pettersson U, Dagälv A, Kjellén L, Lundén A, et al. Serglycin proteoglycans limit enteropathy in *Trichinella spiralis*-infected mice. BMC Immunology. 2016;**17**(1):15. DOI: 10.1186/s12865-016-0155-y

[96] Cvetkovic J, Sofronic-Milosavljevic L, Ilic N, Gnjatovic M, Nagano I, Gruden-Movsesijan A. Immunomodulatory potential of particular *Trichinella spiralis* muscle larvae

excretory-secretory components. International Journal for Parasitology. 2016;**46**(13–14): 833-842. DOI: 10.1016/j.ijpara.2016.07.008

[97] Ding J, Bai X, Wang X, Shi H, Cai X, Luo X, et al. Immune cell responses and cytokine profile in intestines of mice infected with *Trichinella spiralis*. Frontiers in Microbiology. 2017;**8**:2069. DOI: 10.3389/fmicb.2017.02069

[98] Bruschi F, Korenaga M, Watanabe N. Eosinophils and *Trichinella* infection: Toxic for the parasite and the host? Trends in Parasitology. 2008;**24**(10):462-467. DOI: 10.1016/j. pt.2008.07.001

[99] Vallance BA, Matthaei KI, Sanovic S, Young IG, Collins SM. Interleukin-5 deficient mice exhibit impaired host defence against challenge *Trichinella spiralis* infections. Parasite Immunology. 2000;**22**(10):487-492. DOI: 10.1046/j.1365-3024.2000.00328.x

[100] Hsieh CS, Heimberger AB, Gold JS, O'Garra A, Murphy KM. Differential regulation of T helper phenotype development by interleukins 4 and 10 in an alpha beta T-cell-receptor transgenic system. Proceedings of the National Academy of Sciences of the United States of America. 1992;**89**(13):6065-6069. PMID: 1385868

[101] Seder RA, Paul WE. Acquisition of lymphokine-producing phenotype by CD4+ T cells. Annual Review of Immunology. 1994;**12**:635-673. DOI: 10.1146/annurev.iy.12.040194.003223

[102] Saraiva M, O'garra A. The regulation of IL-10 production by immune cells. Nature Reviews. Immunology. 2010;**10**(3):170-181. DOI: 10.1038/nri2711

[103] Luttmann W, Knoechel B, Foerster M, Matthys H, Virchow JC, Kroegel C. Activation of human eosinophils by IL-13. Induction of CD69 surface antigen, its relationship to messenger RNA expression, and promotion of cellular viability. Journal of Immunology. 1996;**157**(4):1678-1683. PMID: 8759755

[104] Horie S, Okubo Y, Hossain M, Sato E, Nomura H, Koyama S, et al. 1997. Interleukin-13 but not interleukin-4 prolongs eosinophil survival and induces eosinophil chemotaxis. Internal Medicine. 1997;**36**(3):179-185. PMID: 9144009

[105] Pope SM, Brandt EB, Mishra A, Hogan SP, Zimmermann N, Matthaei KI, et al. IL-13 induces eosinophil recruitment into the lung by an IL-5- and eotaxin-dependent mechanism. The Journal of Allergy and Clinical Immunology. 2001;**108**(4):594-601. DOI: 10.1067/mai.2001.118600

[106] Oettgen HC, Geha RS. IgE regulation and roles in asthma pathogenesis. The Journal of Allergy and Clinical Immunology. 2001;**107**(3):429-440. DOI: 10.1067/mai.2001.113759

[107] Chomarat P, Banchereau J. Interleukin-4 and interleukin-13: Their similarities and discrepancies. International Reviews of Immunology. 1998;**17**(1–4):1-52. DOI: 10.3109/08830189809084486

[108] Gurish MF, Bryce PJ, Tao H, Kisselgof AB, Thornton EM, Miller HR, et al. IgE enhances parasite clearance and regulates mast cell responses in mice infected with *Trichinella spiralis*. Journal of Immunology. 2004;**172**(2):1139-1145. DOI: 10.4049/jimmunol.172.2.1139

[109]   Wang LJ, Cao Y, Shi HN. Helminth infections and intestinal inflammation. World Journal of Gastroenterology. 2008;**14**(33):5125-5132. DOI: 10.3748/wjg.14.5125

[110]   Rogerio AP, Anibal FF. Role of leukotrienes on protozoan and helminth infections. Mediators of Inflammation. 2012;**2012**:595694. DOI: 10.1155/2012/595694

[111]   Akiho H, Blennerhassett P, Deng Y, Collins SM. Role of IL-4, IL-13, and STAT6 in inflammation-induced hypercontractility of murine smooth muscle cells. American Journal of Physiology. Gastrointestinal and Liver Physiology. 2002;**282**(2):G226-G232. DOI: 10.1152/ajpgi.2002.282.2.G226

[112]   Chavez Ruvalcaba F, Chavez Ruvalcaba MI, Hernández Luna CE, Muñoz Escobedo JJ, Muñoz Carrillo JL, Moreno Garcia MA. Evaluation of anti-Trichinella spiralis obtained by sublingual and conventional immunizations with the 45 kDa protein. Acta Biológica Colombiana. 2017;**22**(2):149-156. DOI: 10.15446/abc.v22n2.56809

[113]   Yera H, Andiva S, Perret C, Limonne D, Boireau P, Dupouy-Camet J. Development and evaluation of a Western blot kit for diagnosis of human trichinellosis. Clinical and Diagnostic Laboratory Immunology. 2003;**10**(5):793-796. DOI: 10.1128/CDLI.10.5.793-796.2003

[114]   Muñoz-Carrillo JL, Muñoz-López JL, Muñoz-Escobedo JJ, Maldonado-Tapia C, Gutiérrez-Coronado O, Contreras-Cordero JF, et al. Therapeutic effects of resiniferatoxin related with immunological responses for intestinal inflammation in Trichinellosis. The Korean Journal of Parasitology. 2017;**55**(6):587-599. DOI: 10.3347/kjp.2017.55.6.587

[115]   Chávez Guajardo EG, Morales Vallarta MR, Saldivar Elías SJ, Reveles Hernández RG, Muñoz Escobedo JJ, Moreno García MA. Detección de los cambios Fenotípicos en productos de Ratas Long Evans infectadas con Trichinella spiralis y tratadas con Albendazol. Archivos Venezolanos de Farmacología y Terapéutica. 2010;**29**(2):28-30. ISSN: 0798-0264

[116]   Reveles Hernández RG, Saldivar Elías SJ, Maldonado Tapia C, Muñoz Escobedo JJ, Moreno García MA. Evaluación de la infección de *Trichinella spiralis* en cerdos gonadectomizados, Zacatecas, México. Acta Médica Peruana. 2011;**28**(4):211-216. ISSN: 1728-5917

[117]   Etewa SE, Fathy GM, Abdel-Rahman SA, El-Khalik DA, Sarhan MH, Badawey MS. The impact of anthelminthic therapeutics on serological and tissues apoptotic changes induced by experimental trichinosis. Journal of Parasitic Diseases. 2018;**42**(2):232-242. DOI: 10.1007/s12639-018-0990-2

[118]   Dupouy-Camet J, Kociecka W, Bruschi F, Bolas-Fernandez F, Pozio E. Opinion on the diagnosis and treatment of human trichinellosis. Expert Opinion on Pharmacotherapy. 2002;**3**(8):1117-1130. DOI: 10.1517/14656566.3.8.1117

[119]   Shimoni Z, Klein Z, Weiner P, MoccH PFM. The use of prednisone in the treatment of trichinellosis. The Israel Medical Association Journal. 2007;**9**(7):537-539. PMID: 17710786

[120]   Biddie SC, Conway-Campbell BL, Lightman SL. Dynamic regulation of glucocorticoid signalling in health and disease. Rheumatology (Oxford, England). 2012;**51**(3):403-412. DOI: 10.1093/rheumatology/ker215

[121] Barnes PJ. How corticosteroids control inflammation: Quintiles prize lecture 2005. British Journal of Pharmacology. 2006;**148**(3):245-254. DOI: 10.1038/sj.bjp.0706736

[122] Barnes PJ. Glucocorticosteroids: Current and future directions. British Journal of Pharmacology. 2011;**163**(1):29-43. DOI: 10.1111/j.1476-5381.2010.01199.x

[123] Wullaert A, Bonnet MC, Pasparakis M. NF-κB in the regulation of epithelial homeostasis and inflammation. Cell Research. 2011;**21**(1):146-158. DOI: 10.1038/cr.2010.175

[124] Flammer JR, Rogatsky I. Minireview: Glucocorticoids in autoimmunity: Unexpected targets and mechanisms. Molecular Endocrinology. 2011;**25**(7):1075-1086. DOI: 10.1210/me.2011-0068

[125] Ashwell JD, Lu FW, Vacchio MS. Glucocorticoids in T cell development and function. Annual Review of Immunology. 2000;**18**(1):309-345. DOI: 10.1146/annurev.immunol.18.1.30

[126] Galon J, Franchimont D, Hiroi N, Frey G, Boettner A, Ehrhart-Bornstein M, et al. Gene profiling reveals unknown enhancing and suppressive actions of glucocorticoids on immune cells. The FASEB Journal. 2002;**16**(1):61-71. DOI: 10.1096/fj.01-0245com

[127] Bozic F, Jasarevic A, Marinculic A, Durakovic E, Kozaric Z. Dexamethasone as a modulator of jejunal goblet cells hyperplasia during *Trichinella spiralis* gut infection of mice. Helminthologia. 2000;**37**(1):3-8

[128] Alvarado RM, Meza LE, García ME, Saldívar S, Moreno GA. Hormonal effect on the parasite load in the infection by *T. spiralis* of a murine experimental model. In: Wakelin OP, ed. 9th International Conference Trichinellosis (ICT9); 1996; 107-114

[129] Piekarska J, Szczypka M, Michalski A, Obmińska-Mrukowicz B, Gorczykowski M. The effect of immunomodulating drugs on the percentage of apoptotic and necrotic lymphocytes in inflammatory infiltrations in the muscle tissue of mice infected with *Trichinella spiralis*. Polish Journal of Veterinary Sciences. 2010;**13**(2):233-234. PMID: 20731176

[130] Nilius B, Szallasi A. Transient receptor potential channels as drug targets: From the science of basic research to the art of medicine. Pharmacological Reviews. 2014;**66**(3):676-814. DOI: 10.1124/pr.113.008268

[131] Carnevale V, Rohacs T. TRPV1: A target for rational drug design. Pharmaceuticals (Basel). 2016;**9**(3):52. DOI: 10.3390/ph9030052

[132] Lee YH, Im SA, Kim JW, Lee CK. Vanilloid receptor 1 agonists, capsaicin and resiniferatoxin, enhance MHC Class I-restricted viral antigen presentation in virus-infected dendritic cells. Immune Network. 2016;**16**(4):233-241. DOI: 10.4110/in.2016.16.4.233

[133] Singh S, Natarajan K, Aggarwal BB. Capsaicin (8-methyl-N-vanillyl-6-nonenamide) is a potent inhibitor of nuclear transcription factor-kappa B activation by diverse agents. Journal of Immunology. 1996;**157**(10):4412-4420. PMID: 8906816

[134] Chen CW, Lee ST, Wu WT, Fu WM, Ho FM, Lin WW. Signal transduction for inhibition of inducible nitric oxide synthase and cyclooxygenase-2 induction by capsaicin and related

analogs in macrophages. British Journal of Pharmacology. 2003;**140**(6):1077-1087. DOI: 10.1038/sj.bjp.0705533

[135] Ueda K, Tsuji F, Hirata T, Takaoka M, Matsumura Y. Preventive effect of TRPV1 agonists capsaicin and resiniferatoxin on ischemia/reperfusion-induced renal injury in rats. Journal of Cardiovascular Pharmacology. 2008;**51**(5):513-520. DOI: 10.1097/FJC.0b013e318 16f6884

[136] Gutiérrez-Coronado O, Muñoz-Carrillo JL, Miranda-Beltrán ML, Pérez-Vega MI, Soria-Fregozo C, Villalobos-Gutiérrez PT. Evaluación de la actividad antiinflamatoria de resiniferatoxina en un modelo murino de inflamación inducido por Lipopolicacárido. Revista Latinoamericana de Química [Abstract]. 2012;**39**:287 (Suplemento Especial)

[137] Gamble HR. *Trichinella spiralis* immunization of mice using monoclonal antibody-affinity isolated antigens. Experimental Parasitology. 1985;**59**(3):398-404. DOI: 10.1016/0014-4894 (85)90095-5

[138] Gamble HR. Monoclonal antibody technology in the development of vaccines for livestock parasites. Journal of Animal Science. 1987;**64**(1):328-336. DOI: 10.2527/jas1987. 641328x

[139] Reveles HG, Muñoz EJJ, Saldivar ES, Moreno GMA. Efecto de la inmunoterapia sobre larvas infectantes (LI) de *Trichinella spiralis* implantadas en musculo estriado en modelo experimental. Biotecnología Aplicada. 2000;**17**(2):126. ISSN: 0684-4551

[140] Castañeda CV. Efecto de la inmunoterapia utilizando antígeno soluble total de T. spiralis en cerdos infectados con *T. spiralis.* [thesis]. Unidad Académica de Biología Experimental; 2010

[141] Maldonado Tapia C, Reveles Hernández RG, Saldivar Elías S, Muñoz Escobedo JJ, Morales Vallarta M, Moreno García MA. Evaluación del efecto protector de 2 inmunógenos de *Trichinella spiralis* en ratas Long Evans con modificación nutricional e infectado con *T. spiralis*. Archivos Venezolanos de Farmacología y Terapéutica. 2007; **26**(2):110-114. ISSN: 0798-0264

[142] Wang ZQ, Cui J, Wei HY, Han HM, Zhang HW, Li YL. Vaccination of mice with DNA vaccine induces the immune response and partial potential protection against *T. spiralis* infection. Vaccine. 2006;**24**(8):1205-1212. DOI: 10.1016/j.vaccine.2005.08.104

[143] Crespo JLE, Maldonado TC, Muñoz EJ, Crespo JP, Moreno GA. Implementando la vía sublingual contra Trichinellosis. España: Editorial Académica Española; 2018. p. 95. ISBN: 978-620-2-11982-5, 6202119829